Ninja Air Fryer Recipes for Beginners

The Ultimate Step by Step Guide With Easy, Quick and Delicious Recipes for Learn The Smart Way To Bake And Grill Indoor Effortlessly

By
Megan Buckley

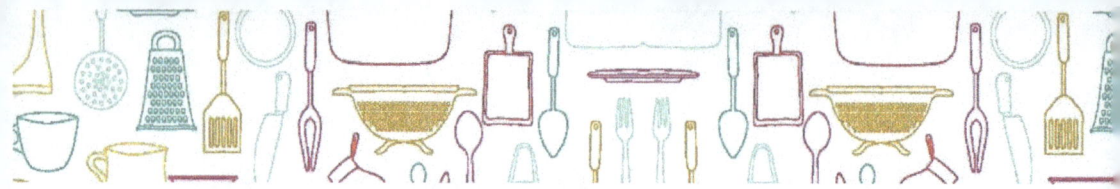

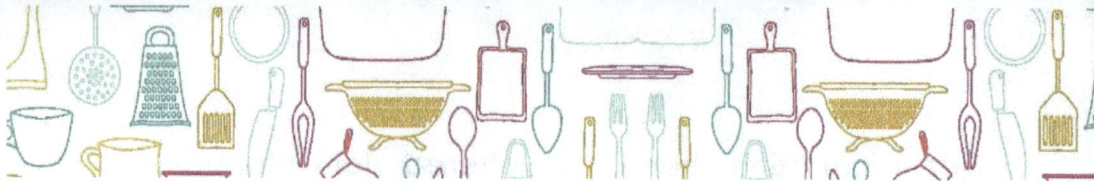

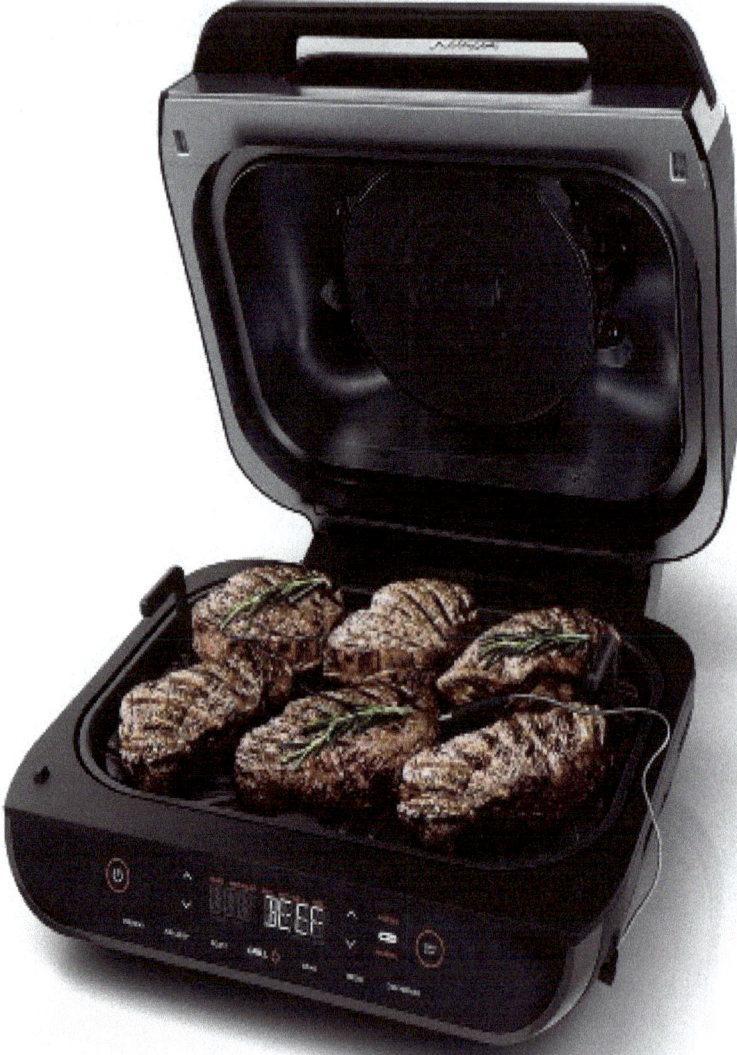

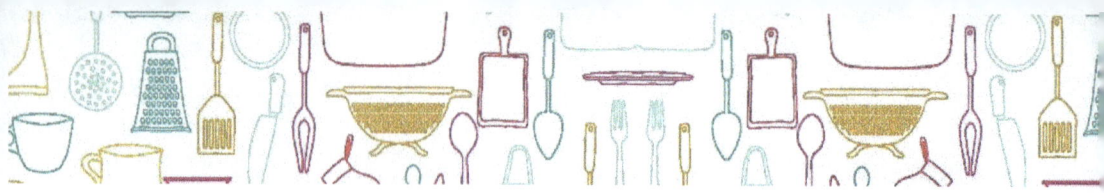

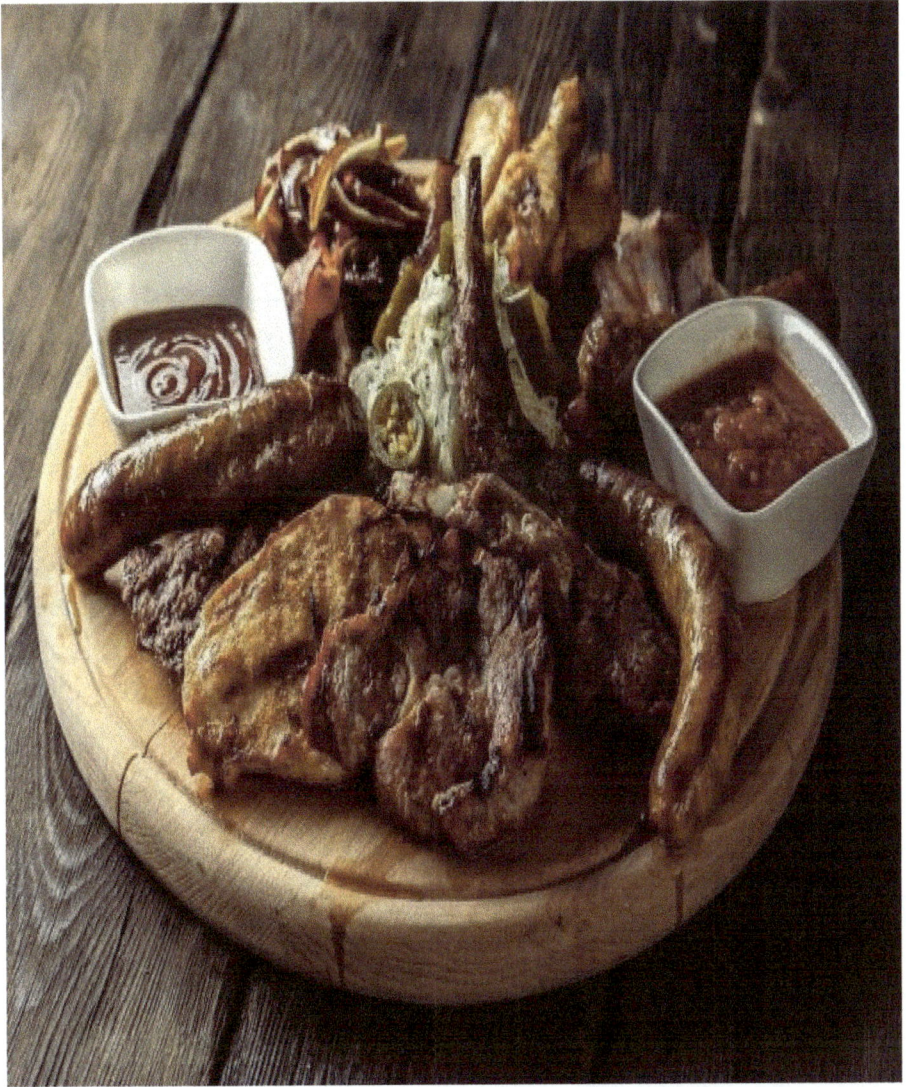

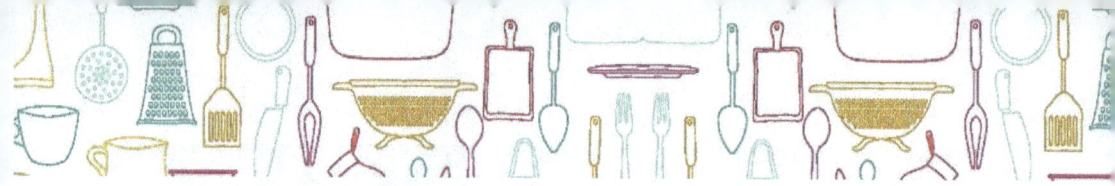

Introduction

The Ninja is a pressure cooker and air fryer that might be used as a microwave, dehydrator, roaster, steamer, and slow cooker.

The principle of Ninja is to provide you with Tender Crisp food from one appliance. It has 2 lids to do this: for tenderness a pressure cooking lid that is detachable and a crisping lid that is non-removable. The new deluxe 8-quart Ninja was released in 2019 by Ninja. A new finish of stainless steel has been included in the new Foodi Deluxe. They also updated the user interface in a big LCD screen and a middle dial for use. It also structures a greater capacity for cooking and a new button for yogurt.

Ninja sent us to test drive both models. Many features still have the same working, despite the display changes, so you can start with the analysis of the original Ninja. It's quick to use the pressure cooker of Ninja. It works comparable to the Instantaneous Pot & other pressure cookers   of   electric.

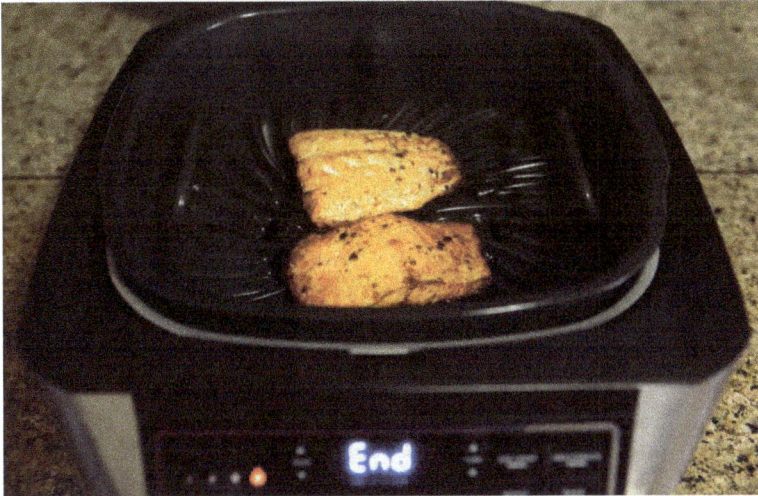

FOODI SPECS

The Original Ninja is well made & robust. There's a really good show window in the Foodi that tells you what's happening in the pot, how much time remains, and tips for the lid to close.

Blue lights revolve in a square on the display while the Foodi pressurizes it and when it has grasped pressure, they stop rotating. It was helpful and quick to follow the Directions manual contained within the Foodi.

A cookbook, and a cooking cheat sheet for frequently cooked products, are included. Included is a Cook and Crisp basket & a rack that is reversible works in high & low positions.

The nonstick ceramic glaze on the pot appears to be well made (some choose ceramic over stainless steel). In crisping up foods, the air fryer ensures great work.

After the time is up, the air fryer counts the time & shuts off, so you don't have to be there to turn it off. The pot is wider and a little shorter than the Instant Pot, so you can easily fit in the pot; four custard cups without stacking them on one another. Best for desserts or for having individual portions. Four ramekins fit comfortably within the Ninja.

What you should know before buying

A large and heavy machine is the Ninja Tender Crisp Pressure Cooker, so you'll need to have a large space vacant to use it. The crisp lid is not removable and hinged (air fryer lid). When using the pressure cooking cover, you need space for the crisp lid to open. The air fryer lid attached ensures you cannot cook under your cabinets on a counter with the Foodi.

The length of the electrical cord of the Foodi is 33", so to use it, you should be closer to the outlet. (The guidelines state that an extension cord should not be used.) The valve of pressure release on it is short & a little harder to manipulate without getting the skin in contact with steam from the Instant Pot.

As its air frying, from the back of the system comes out the hot air, so you should be placing it away from the walls & cabinets. The beep is not very loud and not customizable at the end when your time is up.

Chapter 1: Breakfast and Snack

Breakfast

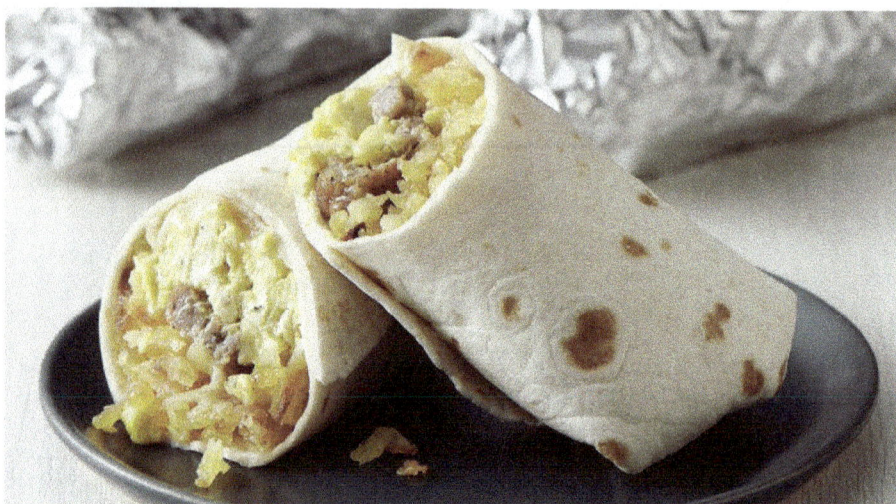

1. Mashed Potatoes

Prep Time: 10 Mins, Total Time: 35 Mins, Serves: 4, Skill: Medium

Ingredients

- Butter salted or unsalted is fine ¼ cup

- Russet potatoes 3 pounds

- Half n half or heavy cream ¾ cup

- Water room temp or cold 3 cups

- Fine grind sea salt divided in recipe 2-3 tbsp.

Directions
- Peel and cut the potatoes into cubes of 1-1½' and apply to the inner container. Add approximately 3 cups of water in. To nearly cover all the potatoes, you only need to have ample water. Add and stir 1 tsp of finely ground salt.

- Put the pressure lid on and seal the valve. Cook at high pressure for 5 minutes and allow the pot to relax naturally for 5 minutes after the time is over. By rotating the valve to Vent, release the residual pressure.

- In the microwave or on the burner, heat the cream or half and half and butter until it is liquid. Do not boil it.

- Scoop out the potatoes and place them in a bowl. Drain the water out of the inner pot and return the potatoes to the pot. Use the sear/sauté on a moderate low until the potatoes are dried and the edge appears white and flaky. I rotate the potatoes a couple of times and sauté for just around 5 minutes. * I used high sear/sauté in my video, but I had some browning so I recommend a lower sauté temp.

- You can either cut the potatoes from the inner pot or put them in a bowl, or you can mash the potatoes right in the ceramic pot if you use the Mix 'N Masher.

- Add 1/4 of the half and half/ice and butter mixture then use a low hand mixer or the Mix 'N Masher to gently blend the liquid into potatoes. You don't want the potatoes to be poured over because they will get too starchy and thick. Continue to apply the butter/half and a half or cream mixture 1/4 at a time until the perfect consistency is the potatoes. Add salt to fit and fold in gently

- If needed, put some pats of butter on top. Serve & Enjoy

2. No Yeast Bread

Prep Time: 5 Mins, Total Time: 85 Mins, Serves: 12, Skill: Difficult

Ingredients

- Olive oil 1 tbsp.

- Medium Russet potato mashed 1, about 1 cup

- Flour divided 4 cups

- Large egg 1

- Baking powder 4 tbsp.

- Sea salt ½ tbsp.

- Butter 1 tsp optional

- Whole Milk 1 cups

Directions

- Peel and dice 1/2"-1" cubes of the Russet Potato. To the inner pot of Ninja, apply 2 cups of water & the diced potatoes. Put on the pressure lid and switch to close the valve. PC up for 2 minutes on big. Unleash the strain instantly. Drain and mash the potatoes with a fork, making sure all the lumps are mashed up. Left to calm aside.

- Combine 3 cups of flour, cinnamon, baking powder, and the mashed potatoes in a medium-sized mixing

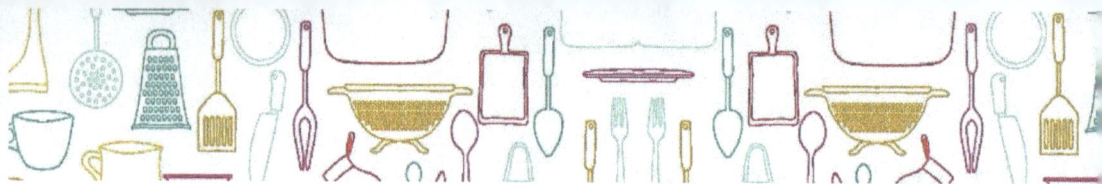

dish. Combine. The mixture is going to be a little bit lumpy, but aim to get pea-size lumps.

- Create a well and add an egg that is gently pounded. Add the milk and the grease. Stir to blend. The dough will start sticky and tacky and a further 1/4-3/4 cup of flour will typically need to be applied. At a time, substitute 1/4 cup. Place it on a floured surface if a shaggy dough ball forms. Preheat the Ninja Foodi for 5-10 minutes to bake/roast @ 375 ° F.

- Simply knead the dough until it fits together. When it is too tacky, apply some starch. Shape a log and put it in the pan for the loaf. Push it down softly enough that it covers the pan's bottom and is also on top. With sharp scissors or a knife, cut large slits in the bread around 2" deep.

- Place the pan in the low position on the rack and place it in the Foodi's inner jar. Pick Bake/Roast at 325 °F and bake for 30 minutes protected (foil or silicone cover). Remove the cover and proceed to bake for another 20 minutes at 325 °F.

- On top, brush some butter and cover the lid of the Tender Crisp. Let the bread stay for another 20 minutes in the Ninja. The center can finish frying. Remove & cool. You can then flip the bread onto a cooling rack or cool it in the pan.

- Cut & Serve.

3. Rolls of Sweet Potato

Prep Time: 15 Mins, Total Time: 100 Mins, Serves: 6, Skill: Easy

Ingredients

- Half or whole milk ¼ cup

- Yeast active dry 1 tbsp.

- Butter 2 tbsp.

- Warm water between 105° f and 115° f 2 tbsp.

- Bread flour 1 ⅔ cup plus extra if needed

- Honey 1 tbsp.

- Sea salt ½ tsp

- Egg 1

- Brown sugar 2 tbsp.

- Sweet potato puree ¼

Directions

- In a tiny bowl, apply the warm water and scatter over the yeast. Enable 5 minutes to flower.

- In the oven, heat the butter & the warm half and half together in a jar for around 30 seconds. To blend, apply the potato mixture & stir. This would push the temperature down because the yeast is not high enough to kill it.

- Add the rice, brown sugar, & salt to a mixing cup or the jar of your stand mixer when the yeast is flowering.

- Add the mixture of yeast, egg, syrup, & butter/ half & half. Turn the mixer to combine ingredients at low to medium altitude using the dough hook or paddle attachment. Combine all ingredients in a big mixing bowl so you have a soft dough, whether you are making this by hand.

- Using a grinder to scrape it back to the center of the flour mix clings to the sides before it gets mixed.

- The dough does not adhere to the fingertips, but it should be very sticky and tacky. Add 1 teaspoon of bread flour & blend again if it sticks to your hands. Repeat it until the dough is tacky, but this doesn't stick to your palms.

- Continue to blend at medium speed with a dough hook for around 5 minutes. That's going to knead the dough. If, during this dough time, the dough gets too sticky, apply another tbsp. of flour and blend again.

- Knead the dough for around 7-10 minutes whether you do this by hand, or until you have a smooth and fluffy dough that does not adhere to your palms.

- Butter your pan and shape a disk with a smooth ball of dough. Place the pan with the dough and cover it with a damp towel. In the lower location, put the pan on the rack, close the Tender Crisp lid and pick the 105 ° F dehydration feature. The reels would be checked in around 30 minutes. If you just don't have the dehydration feature, you can still have evidence in the Ninja Foodi.

- It's time to shape the rolls until the dough is doubled. There is a method that use to shape the rolls and in the recipe.

- In the tray, put the rolls. The gap between rolls would be around 1/2". Cover with a wet towel (and foil or silicone if the dehydration function is used) and prove the rolls again after 30 min or until the scale is doubled. With the rolls, detach the rack.

- Preheat the Ninja for 5 minutes at 350 ° F. Cover the rolls with a foil or silicone cover and put the pan of rolls upon on rack & lower into the Ninja. For 20 minutes, bake covered at 350 ° F.

- Uncover and proceed to bake uncovered at 350 ° F for an extra 3-5 minutes or if they are very brown, lower the temperature to 325 ° F and bake for 3-5 minutes. You may even take a center roll temp and they are finished if it is at least 180 ° F. If needed, brush with melted butter. Allow the rolls to cool slowly, when they cool, they can finish frying.

- Serve & Enjoy

Notes
- If you don't have the dehydration feature, here is how your bread can be evaluated.

- About 5 minutes, put the Ninja to Bake/Roast at 250 ° F. Put the dough in the pan, protected with a wet towel. Place the pan in the lower position on the rack and place it in the inner container. Please ensure the Ninja is switched off and close the lid of the Tender

---

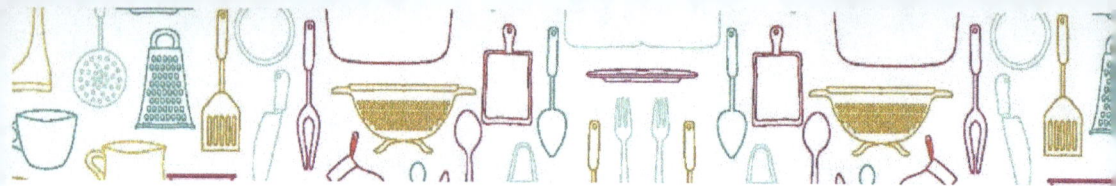

Crisp. The bread would be evidence of the residual heat.

4. Easy Homemade Biscuits

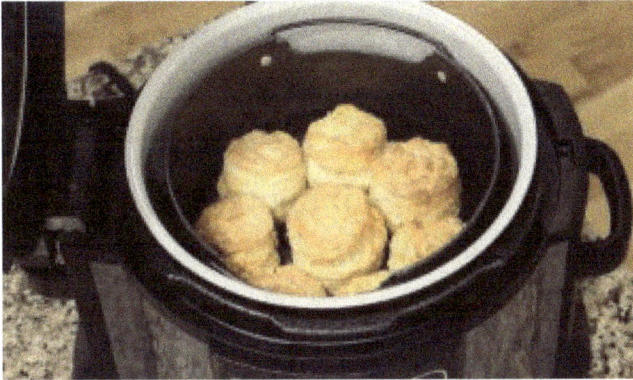

Prep Time: 10 Mins, Total Time: 22 Mins, Serves: 4, Skill: Easy

Ingredients

- 1/4 cup water
- Flour all-purpose 2 cups, chilled
- Greek yogurt plain 1/2 cup, whole fat, unsweetened
- Sea salt fine grind 1/2 tsp
- Butter salted 6 tbsp.
- Baking powder 1 tbsp.
- Granulated white sugar 1 tbsp.

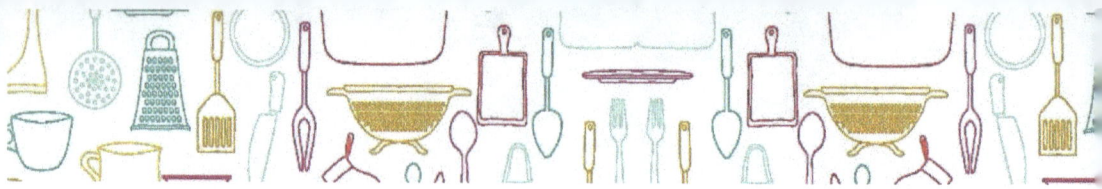

Directions

- On Ninja Foodi, select the Bake function, set the temp to 375°, and set the time to 20 minutes. In a chilled glass dish or metal mixing bowl, combine the flour, baking powder, salt, and sugar.

- Take the butter from the refrigerator and cut it into 1/4 inch pieces with the flour into the bow. Combine the flour and butter with a pastry cutter or fork until it has a rather natural feel.

- Create a well in the center of the mixture of flour/butter and put in the mixture of Greek yogurt and water. Combine the flour mixture & the liquid mixture kindly, using a whisk. You really shouldn't get the dough. For info, see the video.

- Put the mixture onto a floured surface & push down until you have a 4"x 4" slice of dough with your fingertips. Fold the bottom back to the top. Turn 90° and repeat x 5, catching as you go all the loose flour/butter. Make the square bigger any time you click and rotate, just do not go more than 8" x 8".

- Push the dough down softly with your fingertips until it is around 1" thick. Choose a 2" biscuit cutter. Right down, click, and don't twist.

- Gently pull it back together and push it down again to 1" thick after you get as many more biscuits as you can from the dough. You can get at least 8 biscuits. Only 8 can fit in the Ninja.

- You should be able to get 6 to 7 in a circle it around the container of Ninja Foodi, depending on how wide you cut them. Place one in the center and placed the basket in the inner jar.

- Bake for 12 minutes at 375 ° F. Eat and enjoy.

Snack

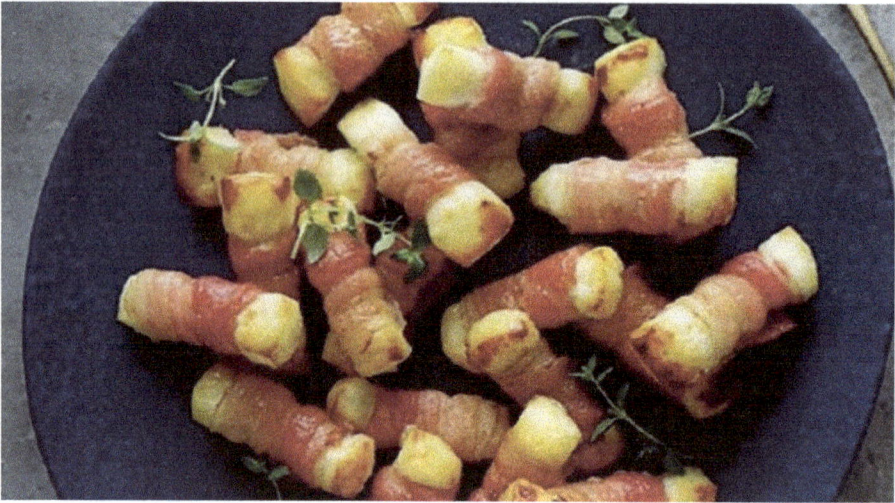

1. Healthy Smokey Baked Beans

Prep Time: 15 Mins, Total Time: 20 Mins, Serves: 3, Skill: Easy

Ingredients

- Chili flakes

- Baby plum tomatoes 100g

- cloves Garlic 2 (crushed)

- Tomato puree 2 tbsp.

- Olive oil 1 tbsp. (for cooking)

- Chopped tomatoes 1 can

- Smoked paprika 1 tbsp.

- Salt & pepper

- Butterbeans 1 can (drained and rinsed)

Directions

- Heat some olive oil over medium flame in a frying pan and add the tomatoes & garlic. Sauté those until the tomatoes tend to burst, then add the puree, tinned tomatoes & seasonings onto them.

- Lower the flame to low/low-medium & allow it to cook and slightly reduce

- Enable this to cool until the sauce has thickened, then pour the blend into the Ninja blender & blitz for a couple of seconds so that you're left with a consistency that is smooth (ish). You should blend this up as much or as little you want.

- Whisk through the butterbeans & adjust some seasonings for taste. Heat up until hot (piping), then serve with a little fresh toast.

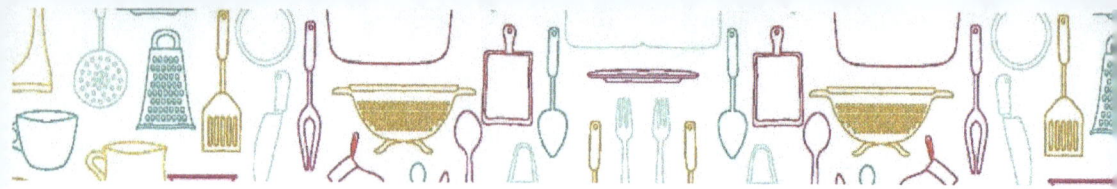

2. Barley Salad with Baby Carrots Pan Fried

Prep Time: 5 Mins, Total Time: 35 Mins, Serves: 2, Skill: Medium

Ingredients

- Olive oil 1 tbsp.

- Cup Dried barley 3/4

- Water 1 1/2 cup

- To taste Salt & pepper

For the salad

- Baby carrots 10

- A handful of Baby tomatoes

- Fresh cucumber 1/3

- Feta cheese 1/2 cup

- A handful sliced Radish

For the carrots

- Fresh herbs

- Olive oil 2 tbsp.

- Sesame seeds

- To taste Salt & pepper

Directions

- To prepare the barley, insert the pot of Multi-Cooker of Ninja with all the ingredients. Combine them well. Gather pressure cooker lid and set the temp to high, and 16 mins of timer.

- Fry the carrots as the barley is cooked, then chop the remainder of the ingredients.

- When barley is prepared, cautiously release the pressure rapidly. Take the lid off when released and left to cool for a few minutes.

- Assemble your salad. You either serve it directly or place it for another day in a lunchbox. It can be stored in the refrigerator for 3 days.

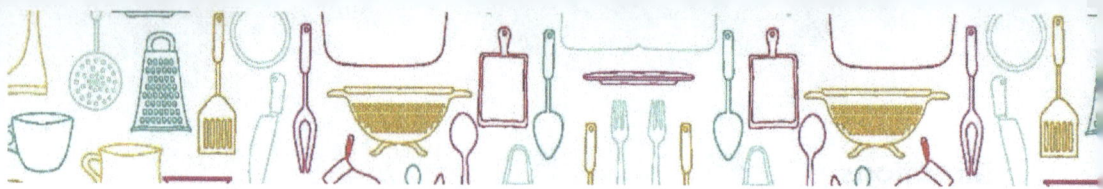

3. Gnocchi with Sage Butter & Walnuts

Prep Time: 2 Mins, Total Time: 15 Mins, Serves: 2, Skill: Easy

Ingredients

- Garlic clove 1 - minced

- Sunflower oil 1 tbsp.

- Sage leaves 6 - julienne cut

- Gnocchi 300g

- Lemon juice 1 tbsp.

- Freshly grated hard cheese 10g

- Butter 30g

- Walnuts 20g

- To taste Salt & pepper

Directions

- Using the pot without the mounted grill plate and crisper basket. Get the lid closed. Choose ROAST, set the temp to 180 ° C, and set the time for 10 mins. To preheat, click START/STOP.

- Put the oil & gnocchi until the machine beeps to show it has preheated. Close the lid to start.

- Open the lid & add butter, garlic, walnuts, sage & season with pepper and salt when the timer shows 5 minutes are left. To continue cooking, stir & close the lid.

- Stir in the hard cheese & lemon juice when the cooking is complete. Instantly serve.

4. Ham and Cheese Noodle Casserole

Prep Time: 30 Mins, Total Time: 30 Mins, Serves: 4, Skill: Difficult

Ingredients

- Nutmeg ¼ tbsp.

- Fine ribbon pasta 300g– cooked

- Pepper ½ tbsp.

- Ham 200g - diced

- Butter 20g - melted

- Salt 1 tbsp.

- Milk 150ml

- Fresh parsley 1 tbsp.

- Eggs 4

Directions

- Place the pot inside the machine and shut the lid. Set the temp to 180 ° C, set the time to 17 mins, and choose BAKE. To commence preheating, click START/STOP

- Put cooked pasta, butter, ham, and parsley in a bowl. Toss it well to spread ham equally in the pasta.

- Stir in the eggs, milk, pepper, salt, & nutmeg in a bowl. Whisk until everything is well integrated.

- Once the machine beeps to show that it has preheated, gently spray the pot with cooking spray. Insert the pasta & then pour the egg mixture into the pot. To start cooking, close the lid.

- Remove the pot when the cooking is finished and allow it to cool down just a bit. Serve as a side or a main.

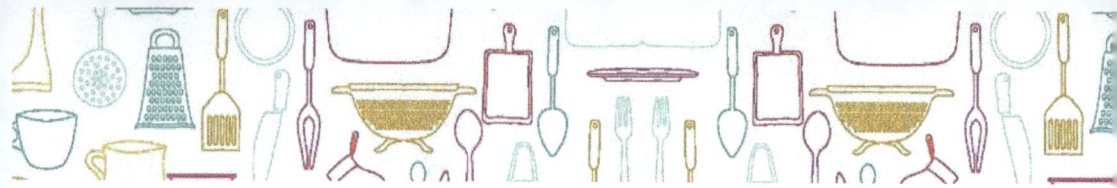

5. Courgette Fries

Prep Time: 15 Mins, Total Time: 25 Mins, Serves: 4, Skill: Easy

Ingredients

- Dairy-free milk 100ml

- Courgettes 3 (cut into fries)

- Breadcrumbs 140g (choose flavored should you wish)

- Plain flour 75g

- Garlic granules ½ tbsp.

- Corn starch 70g

- Salt ½ tbsp.

Directions

- Start the batter by rendering it. Combine the plain flour, salt, corn starch, garlic granules & fat-free milk of your choice.

- In a separate cup, insert the breadcrumbs & then dip each fried courgette in the batter while completely covering it with breadcrumbs.

- Add to the Multi-cooker of Ninja and cook for 10 mins on the air-crisp configuration at 200c.

- Serve with the chosen yogurt-based dip.

Chapter 2: Poultry Mains and Pork, Beef and Lamb Mains

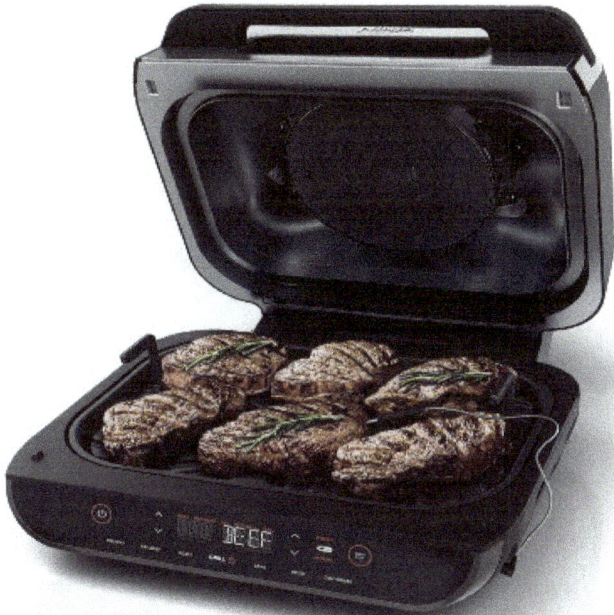

1. Lamb with Mint

Prep Time: 55 Mins, Total Time: 115 Mins, Serves: 4, Skill: Difficult

Ingredients

- Thickening gravy granules 25g

- Half leg of lamb (raw) 1/2 (approximately 1.2kg)

- To taste freshly ground black pepper & salt

- Cloves of garlic 3 (optional - peeled & thinly sliced)

- Rapeseed or vegetable oil 20ml

- Small bunch fresh mint 1 small (approximately 25g) (finely sliced)

Directions

- Put the lamb on the appropriate floor (for the meat). Punch the flesh all over (approximately 30 times) with the point of a sharp knife while utilizing garlic, to create small slits in the beef.

- In each slit, put a slither of garlic that is sliced & seasoning the lamb with fresh black pepper that is grounded and salt.

- Pour, in the pot of the Multi-Cooker of Ninja, 200mls of ice water

- In the Cook and Crisp Basket, put the lamb & place the basket inside the pot (one might have to lean the bone if it's lengthy for the basket)

- Gather the pressure lid and ensure that the valve of pressure release is in the place of the SEAL. Set to HIGH and choose PRESSURE. Configure the period to 32 mins. To commence, pick START/STOP

- Enable pressure to escape naturally for 2 minutes when pressurized cooking is complete. Rapid release of the residual pressure after 2 minutes by carefully changing the pressure release valve to the VENT location. When the machine has done removing pressure, remove the lid.

- Brush the rapeseed/vegetable oil with the lamb

- Please cover the crisp lid. Choose AIR CRISP and set the temp to 200 ° C & set the time to 8 mins. To commence, click START/STOP. Extract basket from the pot when cooking is finished and allow it to settle on a plate, loosely covered with aluminum foil.

- Put the gravy granules in the pot holding the boiling liquid & stir it with a whisk of plastic to incorporate in to create a sauce (or spoon). If required, a bit of water, stock, or one drop of wine may be inserted at this stage. Gather the pressure lid to ensure that the valve of pressure release is in the SEAL location.

- Set to LOW and choose PRESSURE. Set a deadline of 3 mins. To commence, pick START/STOP

- Rapidly relieve the pressure when pressurized cooking is done by shifting the pressure release valve to the VENT location. If the pressure is removed, gently remove the lid.

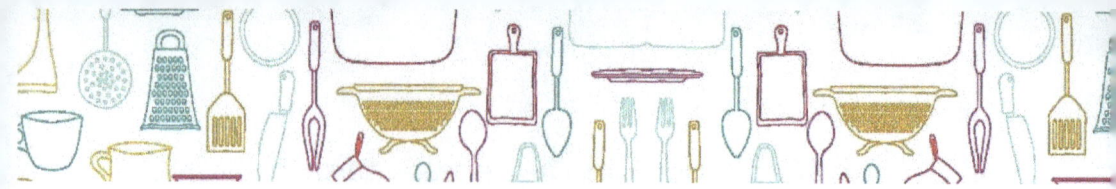

- If it's too thick, swirl the sauce & modify the thickness with a bit more liquid (stock, water, or wine). In a sauce-boat or saucepan, move the sauce via a sieve and put the fresh mint that is finely sliced.

- Carve the resting lamb to serve and put on a warm serving tray. Coat with sauce & serve with freshly steamed seasonal veggies (like dauphinoise) and potatoes.

2. Lamb Kebabs

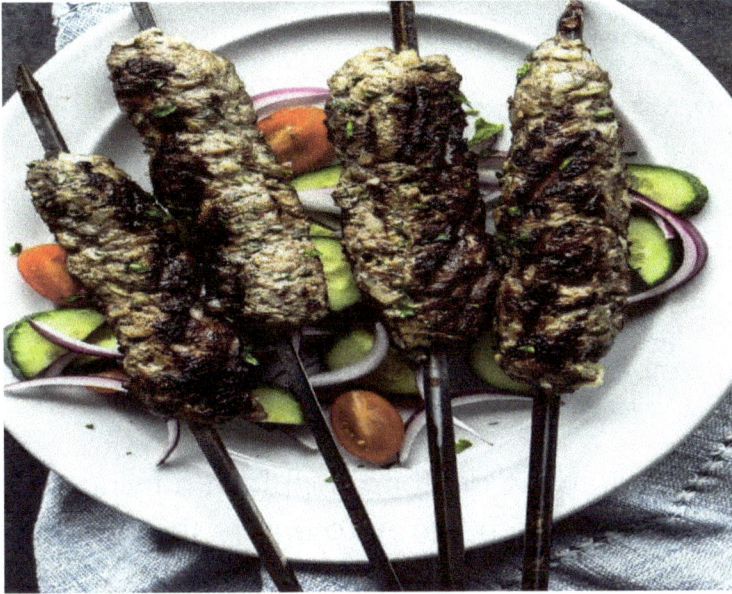

Prep Time: 35 Mins, Total Time: 45 Mins, Serves: 8, Skill: Medium

Ingredients

- Red onion ¼, roughly chopped

- Cumin seeds 2 tbsp.

- Minced lamb 1kg (not too lean)

- Garlic cloves 5

- Green chilies 3

- Coriander stalks 10

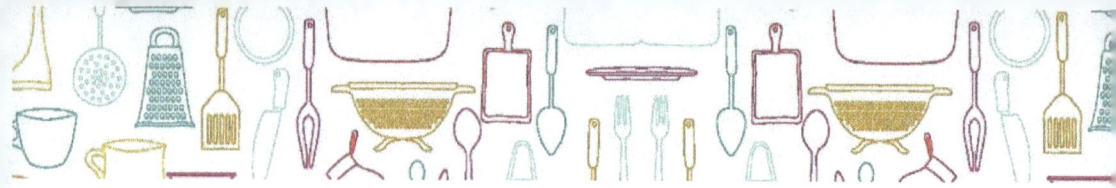

- Ginger crushes 1 inch

- Garam masala 1 tbsp.

- Red chili powder 1 tbsp.

- Black pepper 1 tbsp.

- Cheddar cheese 40g, grated (optional)

- Salt 1.5 tbsp.

- For brushing oil

- Wooden skewers 8, soaked for a few hours

Directions

- Fry the seeds of cumin dry for a minute in a frying pan that is dry on a medium flame. To ensure that they do not burn, monitor them closely. Extract from the pan and add together with the rest of the ingredients to the food processor's bowl.

- Process to merge very rapidly. This is just to get the products together, don't over blend. Conversely, combine by hand,

- Place the mixture into eight balls and then press on the pre-soaked skewers.

- Place them for 30 mins in the freezer. (An optional move, but it makes cooking easier). Place the grill plate in and shut the lid on the Health Grill & Air Fryer of Ninja Foodi.

- Choose Grill, adjust the temp to the maximum setting, and set the timer for 12 mins. Brush with oil on the kebabs and put on the plate of the grill.

- Shut the lid and switch after 6 mins. Check around 10 mins to guarantee that they don't brown too much.

3. Beef Wellington

Prep Time: 15 Mins, Total Time: 35 Mins, Serves: 4, Skill: Medium

Ingredients

- Egg 1, beaten for glazing

- Ready rolled butter puff pastry 320g

- Smooth chicken liver pate 75g

- Olive oil 1 tbsp.

- Ground black pepper to taste

- Filet of beef 500g

Directions

- Crisp basket with a line of baking parchment. Unroll the pastry and break one-third of it off. Roll out a 3rd of the pastry if required, only marginally larger than the beef fillet's length and width. Put it on a crisper basket & prick a fork well. Chill for 15 mins in the freezer.

- In the machine, position the cooking pot and close the lid. Choose BAKE, set the temp to 180 °C, and set the time for 8 mins. To commence preheating, click START/STOP.

- Place the crisper basket in the cooking pot when the machine beeps to show it has preheated. Cover the lid and cook until brown & crisp, or for 8 minutes. Take it out of the oven & leave to cool.

- Heat a tablespoon of oil on high heat in a pan. Seasoning beef with black pepper freshly grounded, then position in the pan & sear on each side for 1 minute until browned throughout. Left to cool aside.

- On Top of the pastry position the cooled meat. With pate paste, cover the top & sides. Layover the top of the leftover rolled out pastry, tucking it to secure under the pastry foundation. To achieve a diamond effect, slice any drippings into lengths & lay over the top, brushing the pastry with the beaten egg all over.

- Link a probe to a device. In the machine, put the pot and close the lid. Set the temp to 180 °C, select ROAST, then choose PRESET. Choose BEEF, using the arrows at the right side of the screen and then the arrows at the left to choose MED RARE or the desired doneness. To commence preheating, click START/STOP.

- While the device is preheating, insert the probe into the beef core (see directions for the positioning of the probe)

- When the machine beeps to show that it has preheated, put the beef in the pot in the crisper basket. Close the probe cord's lid.

- Use oven gloves to detach the probe from beef if the device beeps to warn that the beef has been almost cooked. Then switch wellington beef to a board & enable to rest before serving for up to 10 mins.

4. Spicy Beef Jerky

Prep Time: 10 Mins, Total Time: 20 Mins, Serves: 4, Skill: Easy

Ingredients

- Pepper ½ tbsp.

- Flank steak 200g– thinly sliced into 2mm thick slices

- Salt ½ tbsp.

- Chili flakes ½ tbsp.

- Cayenne pepper ½ tbsp.

Directions

- Add all the ingredients to a medium-sized bowl and blend properly. Spread the slices of meat on a chopping board & pound out very lightly. Which would make the spice fit through the meat and gently tenderize it. The slices of meat should be around 1mm thin when completed.

- Install the pot and in the lower place put the rack that is reversible in the pot. On the rack Place half the beef and then put the top tier dropping it via reversible rack handles. Shut the crisp lid and insert the remainder of the beef.

- Set the duration to 8 hours by choosing DEHYDRATE. To commence, click START/STOP.

- Preserve up to a week in an air-tight container.

5. Chicken, Mushroom, Leek, & Pie of Puff Pastry

Prep Time: 25 Mins, Total Time: 65 Mins, Serves: 4, Skill: Difficult

Ingredients

- Light olive oil 2 tbsp.

- Egg yolk 1

- Skinless, boneless chicken thighs 300g, cut into chunks of 2cm

- Chunky smoked bacon/pancetta lardons 60g

- Chopped tarragon 1 1/2 tbsp.

- Chestnut mushrooms 300g

- Large leek 1, cut into 1 1/2cm slices

- Chopped flat parsley 1 1/2 tbsp.

- Sprigs thyme 4, leaves picked

- Ready-made béchamel/white sauce 275ml

- Dijon mustard 2 tbsp.

- Chopped chives 1 1/2 tbsp.

- All-butter puff pastry 200g (preferably in a block), kept fridge cold

- To taste, salt & pepper

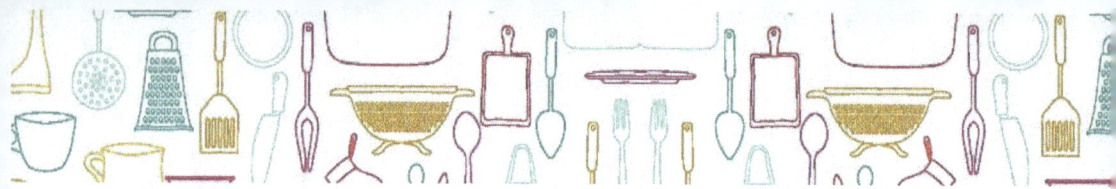

Directions

- Put the basket of air fryer in and close the machine's door.

- At 200 ° C, select an Air Fry.

- Set a timer of 20 mins. Insert chicken wings to guarantee they don't really smoke and turn after 5 minutes.

- Mix all ingredients in a bowl for marinade & whisk them together.

- Toss the wings into the marinade.

- Put the wings again to the air fryer on the grill setting at 260 C for a minute or two.

6. Chicken Couscous Bowl

Prep Time: 10 Mins, Total Time: 25 Mins, Serves: 2, Skill: Easy

Ingredients

- Water 120ml

- Tomato puree 2 tbsp.

- Vegetable stock cube 1/2

- Couscous 120g

- Siracha sauce 1 tbsp.

- Chicken breasts, sliced 2

- Oil 1 tbsp.

- Tomatoes 2, diced

- Paprika 1 tsp

- Garlic powder 1 tsp

- Onion 1, peeled & diced

- Salt & pepper

- Bell pepper 1, deseeded & diced

- For garnishing parsley feta & cheese

Directions

- Boil 120 ml of water and transfer some of the vegetable stock. Stir until the stock dissolves. In a bowl put the couscous and pour over it with vegetable stock. Cover and set the bowl on the side.

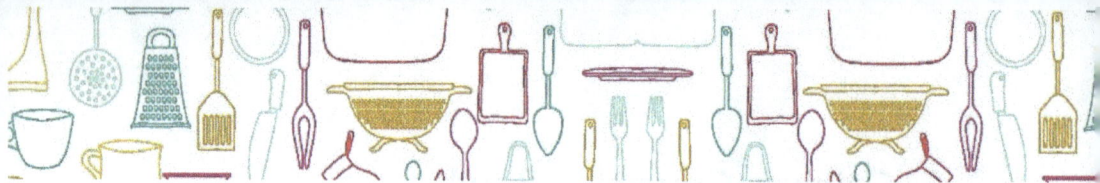

- Ensure that a pot is placed, but remove the grill plate. Choose ROAST, set the temp to 200 ° C, and set the timer for 15 mins. To commence preheating, click START/STOP.

- Mix the chicken, paprika, oil, garlic powder, pepper, and salt together in a dish.

- Once the device beeps to signal that it has preheated, insert the seasoned chicken & close the lid to start cooking.

- Open the cover & put bell pepper, tomatoes and onion when 10 mins are remaining on the timer. To keep cooking, close the lid.

- Insert Siracha, tomato puree & already cooked couscous & mix well when there are 3 minutes left on the timer.

- Stir in the parsley & garnish with the feta cheese until the cooking phase has been finished. Serve it hot.

7. Roasted Broccoli with Breaded Chicken Tenders

Prep Time: 15 Mins, Total Time: 27 Mins, Serves: 4, Skill: Medium

Ingredients

- Kosher salt 1 tsp

- Plain flour 120g

- Medium eggs 2, beaten

- Large broccoli crown 1, cut into florets of 5cm

- Water 125ml plus 2 tbsps. divided

- Uncooked chicken tenderloins 450g

- Bread crumbs 250g

For serving

- Ranch dressing

- Ketchup

- Honey mustard

Directions

- Position flour in a bowl/plate that is shallow. In another cup, put the eggs & 2 tsp. of water and whisk to mix. Place the bread crumbs to a third cup or dish.

- Working in tiny batches, toss the chicken in the flour. Tap off the surplus, then cover the chicken with the egg mixture. Move chicken to the crumbs to cover equally, tossing well. Set them aside.

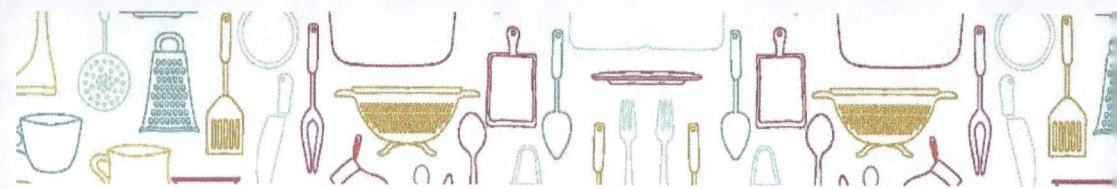

- Place the broccoli in the pot with 125ml of water. Assemble the pressure lid to maintain the SEAL location of the pressure release mechanism.

- Set to LOW and pick PRESSURE. Set the period to 0 minutes, long enough to partly cook the broccoli, the time the machine takes to pressurize. To commence, click START/STOP.

- When the pressure cooking is over, the pressure is easily released by shifting the valve of pressure release to the VENT location. When the machine has done removing pressure, gently remove the lid.

- Put the Reversible Rack over the broccoli in the pot to guarantee that it is at the highest place. Lay chicken tenders on a rack, without overlapping, spaced out equally.

- Cover the crisping lid. Choose the BAKE/ROAST option, set the temp to 180°C, & set the time to 12 mins. To commence, click START/STOP.

- Season the chicken & broccoli with salt & eat with your preferred condiments when the cooking is finished.

8. Chicken Paella

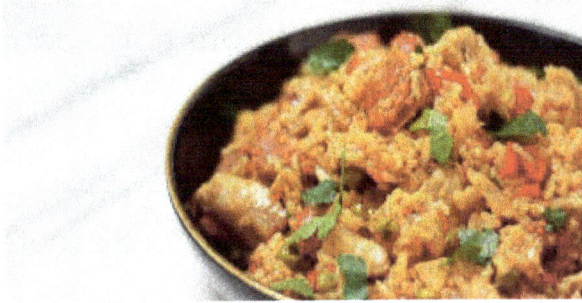

Prep Time: 4 Mins, Total Time: 25 Mins, Serves: 4, Skill: Easy

Ingredients

- Olive oil 1 tbsp.

- White wine 75ml

- Onion 1, diced

- Hot vegetable stock 700ml

- Garlic clove 1, chopped

- Chicken thighs 300g, chopped

- Paella rice 300g

- Chorizo 100g, chopped

- Smoked paprika 1/2 tsp

- Frozen peas 150g

- Chopped rosemary 1 tsp

- Red pepper 1, diced

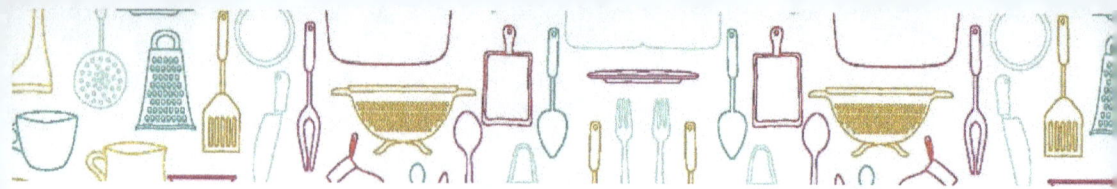

Directions

- Choose SEAR/SAUTÉ & choose HIGH. Click START/STOP and give 3 minutes for the pot to get hot. Add oil & onions, combine and simmer for 2-3 minutes with a wooden spoon.

- Connect the ginger, chicken thighs & chorizo & cook until all the chicken has become white for 3 minutes.

- Connect paprika, red pepper, rosemary, frozen peas, stock, rice, and wine to the remaining ingredients and mix well. Select START/STOP.

- Safe the pressure lid & switch to the SEAL turn the valve of pressure release.

- Choose the PRESSURE button & set it to 7 minutes on HIGH. To commence, click START/STOP.

- Enable the pressure to escape naturally for 2 minutes when the pressure cooking is done. Rapid release of the pressure after 2 minutes by turning the valve of pressure release to the VENT location. When the machine has done removing pressure, gently remove the lid.

- Immediately serve.

9. Curry Chicken Skewers & Mint Dip

Prep Time: 70 Mins, Total Time: 80 Mins, Serves: 4, Skill: Difficult

Ingredients

- Chicken breasts 4 (cut into cubes of 2x2cm)

- Pinch pepper and salt

- Tomato puree 1 tbsp.

- Lemon juice 1 tbsp.

- Rapeseed oil 1 tbsp.

- Garlic powder 1 tbsp.

- Cucumber 1/2– grated

- Turmeric 1/4 tbsp.

- Garam masala 1/4 tbsp.

- Ginger powder 1/4 tbsp.

- To taste salt & pepper

- Chili powder 1 tbsp.

- Plain yogurt 150g

- Mint leaves 10 (finely chopped)

- For garnish coriander leaves

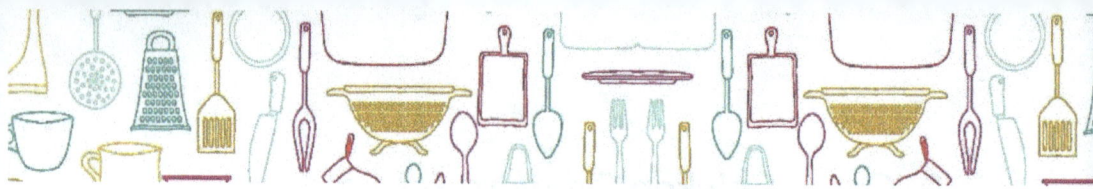

Directions

- Mix the chicken with the tomato puree, the oil, and all the spices in a dish. Set aside and let it marinate for an hour.

- Combine the yogurt, lemon juice, mint, salt & pepper with the grated cucumber, & refrigerate until consumed.

- In the machine, insert the grill plate and close the cover. Choose GRILL, set the Peak temperature, and set the time to 10 mins. To commence preheating, click START/STOP

- Gather the skewers till they're complete when the machine is preheating,

- Position skewers on the plate of the grill when the machine beeps to signal it has preheated. Cover the lid & cook for about five minutes.

- Rotate the skewers after 5 mins and continue to cook.

- Serve hot with the mint dip when the cooking is finished.

10.   Butter Chicken

Prep Time: 2 Mins, Total Time: 25 Mins, Serves: 4, Skill: Easy

Ingredients

- Boneless chicken thighs 1lb
- Chopped tomatoes 1 tin
- Double cream 115ml
- Garam masala 1 tsp
- A pinch of Fenugreek leaves
- Black pepper 1/4 tbsp.
- Garlic cloves 6
- Smoked paprika 1 tbsp.
- Turmeric powder 1 tbsp.
- Ground cumin 1 tbsp.
- Red chili powder 1/2 tbsp.
- Salt 1 tbsp.
- Ginger 1 inch Chopped coriander

Directions

- Besides the cream, garam masala & chopped coriander, place all the ingredients into Multi-cooker.
- Thoroughly stir.
- Gather the pressure lid to ensure it is set to close the valve. Choose the pressure & set it high.

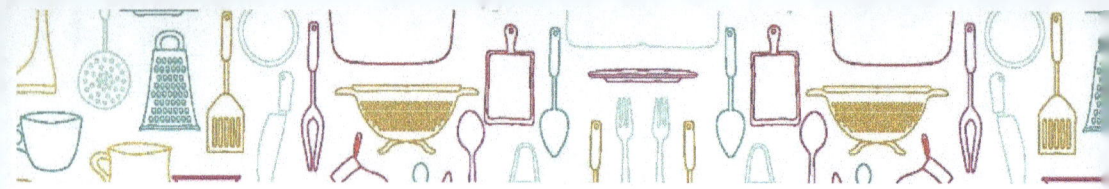

- Set the period for five mins. Hit the start button.

- Once done, the pressure is easily released by slowly shifting the escape valve to the vent.

- Remove the chicken from the pot cautiously and mix the curry with the help of a stick blender.

- Put the chicken back. Setting it too high and select the sauté. Press the Start button and put the double cream.

- For 2 mins, simmer.

- Garnish with coriander & serve with rice, roti, or naan.

11. Chicken Nachos Loaded Upside-Down

Prep Time: 5 Mins, Total Time: 30 Mins, Serves: 4, Skill: Medium

Ingredients

- Chicken breasts 4, (Frozen uncooked skinless)

- Jar of Red salsa 1x450g

- Tortilla chips 110g, divided

- Taco seasoning 2 tbsp.

- Tinned refried beans 435g

- Sea salt 1 tbsp.

- Spring onions, sliced

- Grated cheese 340g

- Sour cream

- Toppings

- Guacamole

Directions

- Position the frozen chicken & salsa to the Multi-cooker of Ninja cooking pot. Gather the pressure lid and check that the valve of pressure release is in the place of the SEAL.

- Selecting PRESSURE to HIGH. Imposed a time limit of 12 mins. To commence, click START/STOP.

- After pressure cooking is over, the pressure is immediately released by shifting the pressure relief valve to the VENT location. When the machine has done removing pressure, remove the lid carefully.

- In the pot Shred the chicken using silicone-tipped utensils. To combine, add refried beans, spice, & taco seasoning and stir well.

- On top of the mixture of chicken, set 1/2 of the tortilla chips equally, and cover the chips with 1/2 of the cheese. Repeat for the leftover tortilla chips with a second layer covered with the leftover cheese.

- Keep the crisping lid close. Choose AIR CRISP, set the temp to 180 ° C, and set the time to 5 mins. To commence, click START/STOP. Add extra time for crispier results.

Cover the nachos with sour cream, guacamole, and spring onions & serve when the cooking is done.

Chapter 3: Soups, Fish and Seafood

1. Hungarian Mushroom Soup

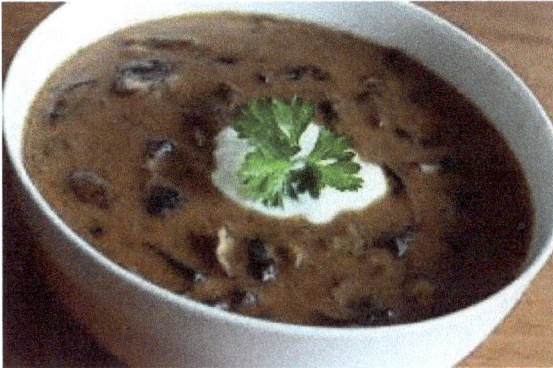

Prep Time: 10 Mins, Total Time: 15 Mins, Serves: 6, Skill: Easy

Ingredients

Ingredients for the OP300

- Fresh parsley 1/2 bunch, chopped

- Butter 60g

- Fresh dill 1 tbsp. Or dried dill 2 tbsp.

- Onion 1 large, diced

- Mushrooms 500g, sliced – any variety you enjoy

- Lemon juice 1 tbsp.

- Flour 3 tbsp.

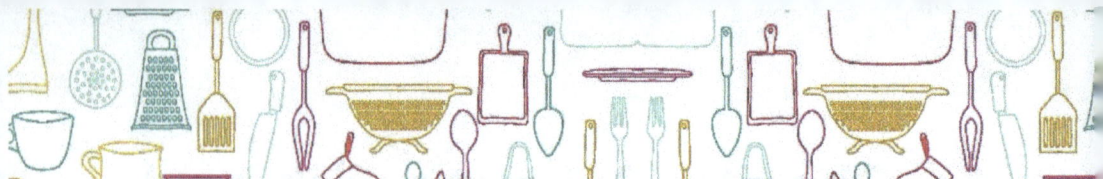

- Paprika 1 tbsp.

- Crème Fraiche 150g

- Vegetable stock 750ml

- Milk 250ml

- Soy sauce 3 tbsp.

- Salt & pepper to taste

Ingredients for the OP500

- Butter 120g

- Fresh parsley 1 bunch, chopped

- Onions 2 large, diced

- Mushrooms 1000g, sliced - any variety you enjoy

- Fresh dill 2 tbsp. Or dried dill 3 tbsp.

- Flour 6 tbsp.

- Paprika 2 tbsp.

- Lemon juice 2 tbsp.

- Vegetable stock 1500ml

- Soy sauce 6 tbsp.

- Crème Fraiche 300g

- Milk 500ml

- To taste salt & pepper

Directions

- Turn the device on, choose SEAR/SAUTÉ and set it to MD:HI. To commence, click START/STOP.

- Add the butter, onions & mushrooms to the food pot and cook for about 5 minutes until the onions are tender.

- Apply the flour and paprika to the mixture and cook for 2 to 3 minutes while stirring.

- Add the soy sauce and milk into the vegetable stock, then combine well.

- Assemble the pressure lid and ensure that the release valve is in the place of the SEAL. Please pick PRESSURE and set HI. Set the time for five minutes. To commence, click START/STOP.

- Enable the device to naturally release pressure for five minutes when pressure cooking is complete, and then manually release pressure by shifting the release valve to the Ventilation position. When the device has finished releasing strain, carefully remove the lid.

- Apply the lemon juice, dill, and parsley to the crème Fraiche. To mix well, stir, then season to taste with salt and pepper.

- Serve right away and enjoy.

2. Green Asparagus Soup

Prep Time: 4 Mins, Total Time: 45 Mins, Serves: 4, Skill: Medium

Ingredients

- Ramson leaves 8 (baerlauch)

- Oil 1 tbsp.

- Green asparagus 350g - halved

- Vegetable stock cubes 2

- Shallot 1

- Water 1l

- To taste salt & pepper

Directions

- To the blender jug, add the oil, the ramson leaves & the shallot.

- CHOP Select.

- SAUTE select.

- Add the rest of the ingredients and choose SMOOTH SOUP.

- Serve cold or hot.

3. Sambar Soup

Prep Time: 10 Mins, Total Time: 45 Mins, Serves: 4, Skill: Medium

Ingredients
Dal
- Water 3 cups

- Toor dal 1 cup

- Turmeric powder 1/2 tbsp.

Vegetable Soup
- Oil 1 tbsp.

- Carrot 1, peeled and diced

- Curry leaves 10 (fresh)

- Drumsticks 8

- Black mustard seeds 1 tbsp.

- Salt 1/2 tbsp.

- Medium tomato 1, diced

- Ghee or oil 1 tbsp.

- Water 3 cups

- Sambar powder homemade 2 tbsp.

- Tempering / tadka (optional)

- Sugar 1 tbsp.

- Tamarind paste 2 tbsp.

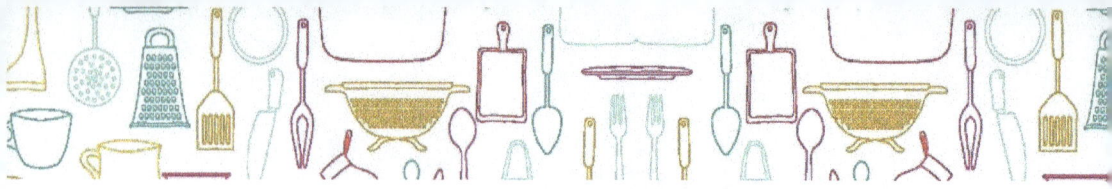

- Red chili powder 1/2 tbsp. (optional)

Directions

- Over medium-high heat, add the ingredient for the dal to a big pot. Simmer until cooked by Dal. That's going to take 30-40 minutes.

- In a blender, add oil, drumsticks, carrots, & salt and pick the sauté.

- Add rest of the ingredients & pick a chunky one.

- Pour the cooked Daal into it and mix it thoroughly.

- Give Tadka (Optional)

- In a pan, warm oil. Add the mustard seeds & curry leaves for a hot one. As soon as the mustard seeds pop, pour the oils over the broth.

4. Mushroom Soup

Prep Time: 10 Mins, Total Time: 10 Mins, Serves: 4, Skill: Easy

Ingredients

- Olive oil 3 tbsp.

- Onions roughly chopped 2

- Double cream 3 tbsp.

- Garlic cloves 2

- Salt & pepper

- Mixed chestnut and button mushrooms 500g, cleaned & chopped

- Milk 200ml

- Vegetable stock 500ml

- To garnish parsley

Directions

- Place in the machine the onions, the garlic, and the mushroom and click the sauté.

- Now add the milk & stock to the soup maker and push the button for a smooth soup.

- Season & decant into bowls until full. Double milk, olive oil, and parsley on top.

5. Haddock Croquettes

Prep Time: 30 Mins, Total Time: 40 Mins, Serves: 4, Skill: Medium

Ingredients

- Dried breadcrumbs 150g

- Fresh breadcrumbs 75g

- Plain flour 100g

- Sherry 2 tbsp.

- Zest of lemon 1

- Uncooked haddock fillets, flaked 500g

- Eggs 3

- White pepper ¼ tbsp.

- Fresh parsley, finely chopped 1 bunch

- Salt ½ tbsp.

- Dried coriander 1 ½ tbsp.

- Rapeseed oil for spraying

Directions

- Put the flaked fish fillets, fresh breadcrumbs, and sherry in a bowl. Mash properly to mix, beat one egg & put chopped parsley, pepper, coriander, salt, and zest of lemon. Mix thoroughly.

- To dip the fish, prepare three dishes. One dish of flour, one dish of breadcrumbs, and one dish of 2 remaining eggs, well beaten. Line a tray of baking with parchment for baking.

- Flour the hands & shape croquettes that are between 5 to 7cm in length, from the mixture. Roll the croquettes into the flour first, then into the egg, and then into the breadcrumbs, and put them on the plate.

- Install the crisper plates into the drawers of zone 1 & 2. Spray the rapeseed oil on a plate. On a crisper plate, position the croquettes & spray the croquettes with oil. Choose AIR FRY, set a temp of 200 °C & set a period of 10 mins. Choose MATCH. To commence, click START/STOP.

- Using silicone-coated tongs for removing the croquettes into a serving dish when the cooking time is completed.

- Serve with tartar sauce, salad and lemon instantly.

6. Tuna, Broccoli, Feta Cheese & Egg Bake

Prep Time: 5 Mins, Total Time: 50 Mins, Serves: 4, Skill: Medium

Ingredients

- Garlic powder 1 tbsp.

- Tin Tuna drained 1 (approximately 100g)

- Feta cheese 100g

- Whole eggs 10

- Pepper & Salt

- Broccoli chopped in small pieces 75g

Directions

- Start by preheating the oven to a degree of 200c.

- Put all of the products in the bowl & pulse until the ingredients are fully blended together using the bowl of the food processor & the plastic blade.

- Pour the egg mixture into the pan and use a loaf tin lined with greaseproof paper, and put it in the oven.

- Bake for 35-45 min or so, pierce in the middle to make sure it is cooked through.

- Before slicing you should wait to cool.

7. Indian Baked Salmon

Prep Time: 3 Mins, Total Time: 10 Mins, Serves: 2, Skill: Easy

Ingredients

- Lemon juice 1 tbsp.

- Oil 1 tbsp.

- Garam masala 1/2 tbsp.

- Red chili powder 1 tsp

- Pieces Salmon 2

- Turmeric powder 1/2 tbsp.

- Crushed ginger 1 tbsp.

- Cloves of garlic 3

- Salt (Pinch)

Directions

- Clean the fillets with a paper towel.

- Drizzle the fish oil on all sides of the fish properly.

- Rub on all sides of the rest of the ingredients onto the fish.

- Turn your Air Fried Multi-cooker of Ninja to 200 degrees & cook it for 5-6 minutes. After 5 minutes, review and raise the time if required.

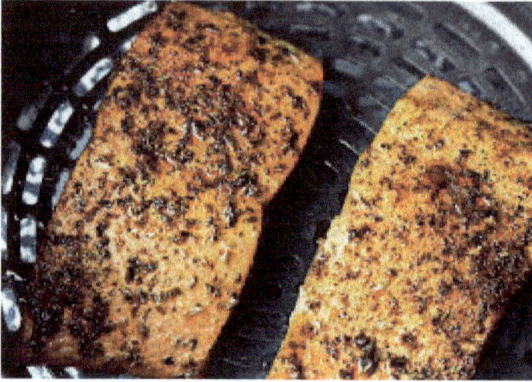

8. Sweet and Spicy Salmon

Prep Time: 2 Mins, Total Time: 15 Mins, Serves: 3, Skill: Easy

Ingredients

- Lemon 2 tbsp.
- Salmon fillets 3 (200g each)
- Oil 2 tbsp.
- Soft light brown sugar 1 tbsp.
- Salt 1/2 tbsp.
- Garlic cloves 4
- Cumin powder 1 tbsp.
- Tamarind 1/2 tbsp.
- Red chili powder 1/2 tbsp.

- Turmeric 1/4 tbsp.

Directions

- To make a marinade, mix all the ingredients together except the salmon.

- Marinate the salmon for 1 hour in mixture.

- The Ninja Fitness Grill and Air Fryer Preheat

- Put the salmon fillets high on the grill plate and close the door.

- For 10 - 15 min, cook. Check in the middle & change the temperature and time if it is too fast to grill.

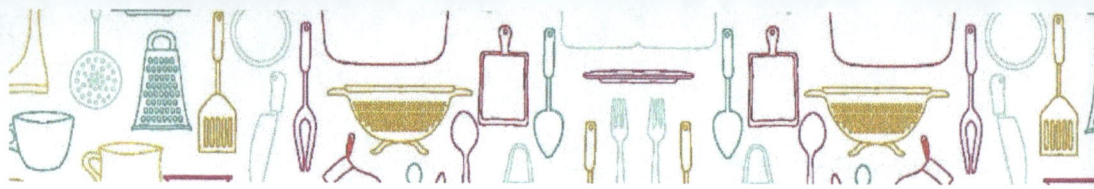

6. Sea Salt Focaccia

Prep Time: 35 Mins, Total Time: 8 Hrs 25 Mins, Serves: 8, Skill: Difficult

Ingredients
Ingredients for the AG301

- Water 225ml

- Flaked sea salt A pinch

- Strong plain flour 350g

- White wine 60ml (or use all water)

- Extra virgin olive oil 3 tbsp. (divided, plus a little extra for greasing)

- Dried yeast 1 tbsp.

- Fine sea salt 1 1/4 tbsp.

Ingredients for the AG551

- Flaked sea salt for sprinkling

- Strong plain flour 400g

- Tepid water 250-300ml

- Sachet fast action/easy bake yeast 1

- Extra virgin olive oil 3 tbsp. (divided)

- Salt 1 1/4 tbsp.

Directions

- In a bowl, combine the yeast, flour, sea salt, and 2 tbsp. of olive oil, wine, and water. For around one to two minutes, mix it approximately by one-handed kneading operation to ensure everything is well blended. The dough's going to be sticky.

- Cover the bowl with a film of cling and put it in the refrigerator to prove for at least 8 hours or maybe up to 24 hours. (Prove at room temp for around 2 hours or before doubled in size for the rapid method.)

- About 2 hrs before you intend to bake focaccia, take out the dough from the fridge.

- Cover the crisping basket on the sides with baking parchment about 5 cm up. There's no reason for it to be neat & perfect. Lightly oil the parchment and your hands. Take the dough & put it in the crisp basket, loosely stretching it out to the corners. (As it indicates, it can disperse more & fill the basket).

- Cover the crisp basket with a film of cling and leave to be checked for at least 2-2 1/2 hours at room temp. (If the faster measurement approach is used, the second test would take around 30 mins or till the volume is doubled).

- Mix the leftover 1 tbsp. of olive oil along with 1 tbsp. of water when you are about to bake focaccia, then drizzle it across the focaccia surface. By pressing the fingertips in, use both hands to dimple dough on the board all over. Sprinkle with flakes of sea salt & any extra toppings you may need.

- Making sure the machine has the pot inserted & close the lid. Choose BAKE, set the temp to 190 °C, and set the time for 25 minutes. To commence preheating, click START/STOP.

- Position the crisping basket in the pot & close the lid when the machine beeps to signal it has preheated. After 18 minutes, check the focaccia. When tapped, it can sound hollow if fried & should be well browned on top. Raise the crisping basket gently out of the machine when focaccia is cooked & extract the focaccia on the parchment of baking. Move the focaccia, extracting the parchment from beneath it, onto a cooling shelf. Before consuming, cause it to cool.

7. Salt and Pepper Chips

Prep Time: 5 Mins, Total Time: 35 Mins, Serves: 4, Skill: Medium

Ingredients
- Chicken stock 125ml

- Organic potatoes 4 cut into ⅙

- Sea salt ½ tsp

- Olive oil 1 tbsp.

- Ground black pepper 1 tbsp.

For the spicy garlic mayo
- White wine vinegar ½ tbsp.

- Mayo 3 tbsp.

- Garlic powder 1 tbsp.

- Siracha 1 tbsp.

Directions
- Pour the stock of chicken into the pot from the French Dressing Chicken, drop potatoes in the cook and crisp basket & lower it in the pot. Place the pressure lid on to ensure that the valve is in place of the seal. Then push and adjust the pressure to medium. Set timer to 3 mins, then. Move the valve of pressure release to the location of the vent when 3 mins are over. Remove the lid carefully when pressure has been removed.

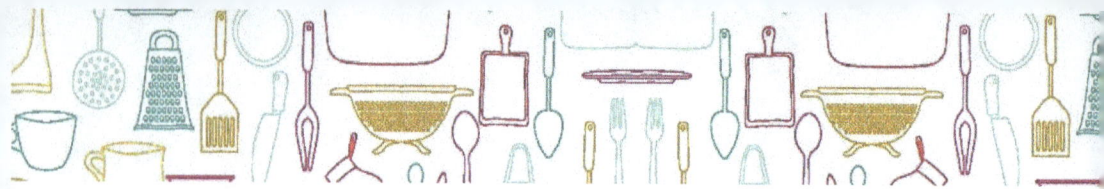

- Now spill the oil over the potatoes uniformly and mix the salt & pepper with it. Cover the crisping lid & at 200c, choose air crisp. For 30 mins, set the timer. Press start. After 15 minutes, normally look & give them a switch to keep cooking till they are crisp enough to leave you satisfied.

- It's pretty simple if you want to put Spicy Garlic Mayo. Bung the all ingredients into a bowl and mix.

8. Grilled Watermelon

Prep Time: 5 Mins, Total Time: 7 Mins, Serves: 4, Skill: Easy

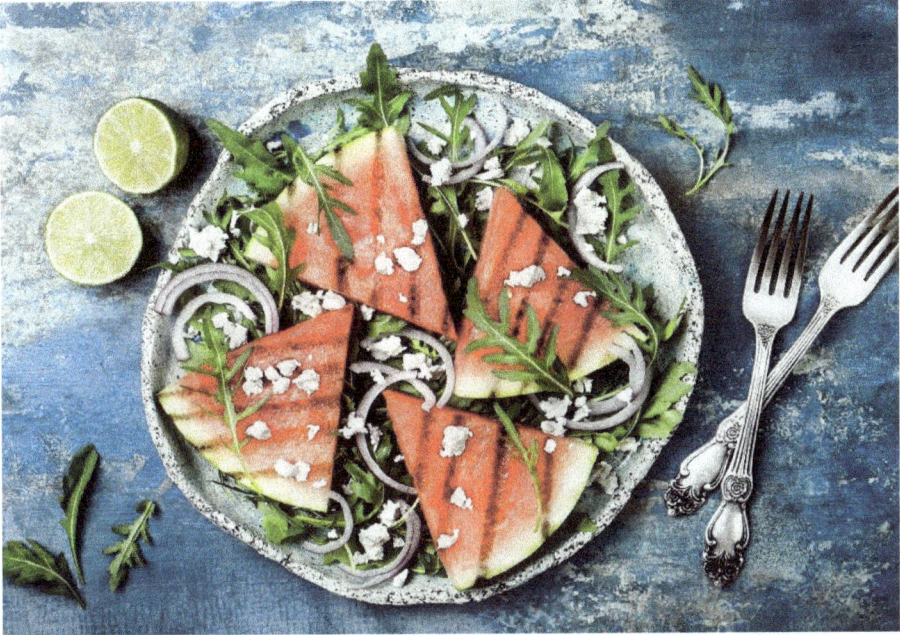

Ingredients

- White sugar 1 tbsp.

- Watermelon 6 slices around 7.5cm

Directions

- Place the grill plate in the Health Fryer & Air Grill of Ninja and shut the lid. Choose GRILL, set the Peak temperature, and set the time to 2 mins. To commence preheating, click START/STOP

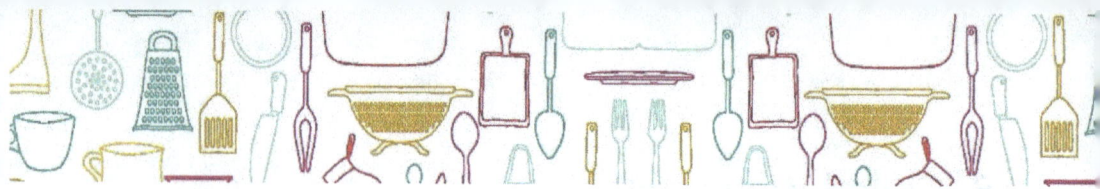

- When the machine preheats, watermelon slices are liberally seasoned on both sides with white sugar.

- Place the watermelon on the grill plate when the machine beeps to show it has preheated. To maximize contact with the grille, press down softly. Without turning, shut the lid & grill for 2 mins.

- Serve directly when the cooking is done. TIP: To give a kick to these slices of watermelon, apply 2 teaspoons of chili powder & 1 lime zest in the sugar before you season the fruit.

Chapter 4: Vegetarian, Vegan Recipes and Special Recipes

If you are in for some beautiful, leafy greens and juicy vegetables then this chapter is all that you will be striving for. In this chapter, you will learn some very healthy and special, easy to cook, and machine-friendly recipes. All these recipes are gathered with taking full care of the beginners.

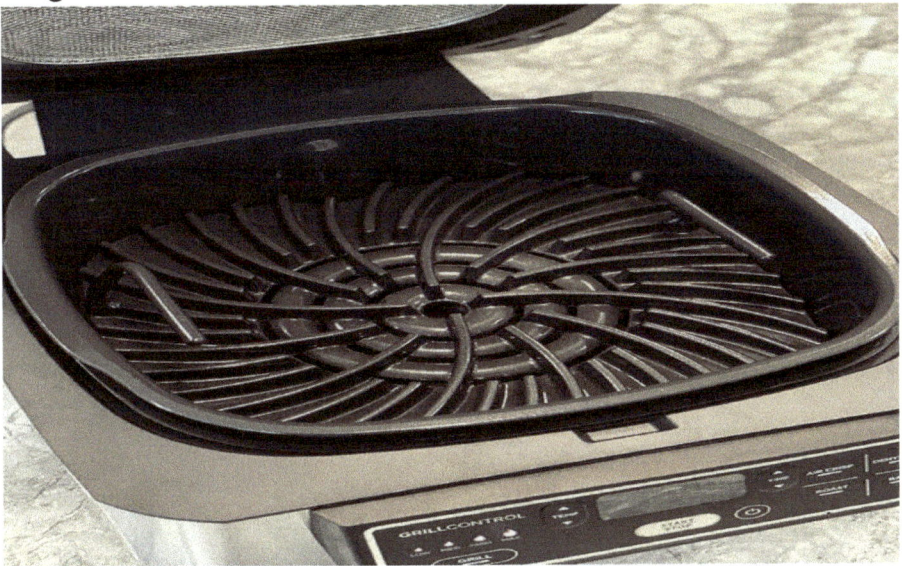

1. Chickpea & Beetroot Koftas

Prep Time: 20 Mins, Total Time: 2o Mins, Serves: 2, Skill: Easy

Ingredients

- Cooking spray
- Chickpeas 200g (drained)
- Pickled beetroot 40g (drained)
- Salt and pepper to taste
- Shallot 1 - diced
- Vegan breadcrumbs 20g
- Coriander 1 tsp - freshly chopped
- Garlic cloves 1
- Cumin ¼ tsp
- Cayenne pepper ½ tbsp.
- Cinnamon ¼ tsp

Directions

- In a blender, put all ingredients. Blend once well mixed, but still with tiny chunks left
- In the machine, insert the grill plate and close the lid. Click the GRILL tab, set the temp to HIGH, & set the time to 10 mins. To commence preheating, click START/STOP

- Divide the chickpea mix into 4 equal sections when the machine is preheating and shape mini loaves from around skewers.

- When the machine beeps to show that it has preheated, with cooking spray, spray on the grill plate and insert the koftas. To start cooking, close the lid.

- The koftas are flipped after 5 min to obtain grill marks on both sides. To continue cooking, close the lid.

- Serve with grilled veggies or salad right away.

2. Celeriac Soup

Prep Time: 2 Mins, Total Time: 45 Mins, Serves: 4, Skill: Difficult

Ingredients

- Olive oil 2 tbsp.

- To taste salt & pepper

- Small onion 1 (roughly chopped)

- Wholegrain mustard 1 heaped tbsp.

- Leek ½ (roughly chopped)

- Hot vegetable/ vegan stock 750ml

- Stick celery 1 (roughly chopped)

- Pear 1 (peeled and quartered)

- Peeled celeriac 500g, cut into 2.5cm pieces

Directions

- In the jug of the Blender & Soup Maker of Ninja, put onion, olive oil, leek & celery, close the lid and choose CHOP.

- Select SAUTE once the process has ended,

- Add to the jug the celeriac, pear & veg stock, lock the jug's lid and choose SMOOTH SOUP

- When the SMOOTH SOUP setting is over, insert the wholegrain mustard in the jug carefully & pulse to blend quite briefly. To taste, insert salt & pepper.

3. Panko Broccoli Bites

Prep Time: 10 Mins, Total Time: 20 Mins, Serves: 2, Skill: Easy

Ingredients

- Chopped chives to taste

- Large head broccoli 1 (cut into florets)

- A pinch salt

- Dairy-free milk 220ml

- Soy sauce 1 tbsp.

- Plain flour 80g

- Juice of ½ lime

- Sriracha 1 tbsp.

- Panko bread crumbs 120g

- Corn starch 75g

- Vegan mayo to taste spicy

Directions

- Start the batter by making it. Mix the flour, dairy-free milk, corn starch, sriracha, lime juice, salt & soy sauce together.

- In a bowl empty the bread crumbs of panko & dip each floret of broccoli in the batter before completely covering it with breadcrumbs.

- Add to your Multi-Cooker of Ninja Foodi, and cook for 10 minutes at 200C on-air crisp mode.

- Serve with vegan spicy mayo & chopped chives

4. Chana Saag (Spinach & Chickpeas)

Prep Time: 5 Mins, Total Time: 45 Mins, Serves: 4, Skill: Medium

Ingredients

- Garam masala 1/2 flat tbsp.

- Oil 2 tbsp.

- Chickpeas 2 x 400g tins (drained)

- Onions 4 (diced)

- Plum tomatoes 400g tin

- Garlic cloves 2

- Ginger 2 inch

- Red chili powder 1-2 tbsp.

- Ground coriander 2 tbsp.

- Turmeric powder 1/2 tbsp.

- Ground cumin 1 tsp

- To taste salt

- Baby Spinach 4 handfuls

Directions

- In a pot, add oil over high heat & add the onions once heated. Sauté the onions with a dose of salt for 10 minutes, until golden brown.

- Meanwhile, with a water's splash in the blender, purée the garlic and ginger. Stir in and simmer for about 5 minutes with the onion.

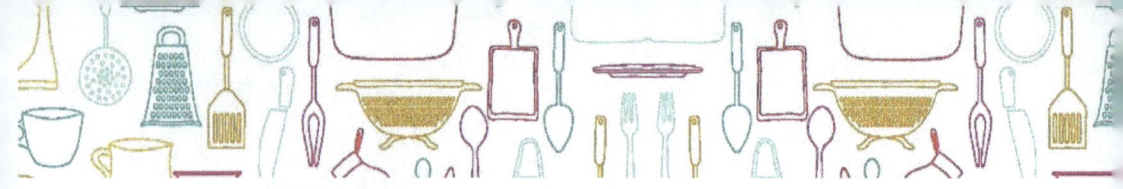

- Apply the coriander, cumin, chili & turmeric & stir for one minute. If the mixture tends to get stuck to the base of the pot, insert a tbsp. of hot water and blend.

- In the blender Purée the plum tomatoes and add 100ml of water to the masala.

- Reduce the heat after boiling and allow 15 mins to simmer.

- Put the chickpeas in & stir. Before folding the spinach in, cook chickpeas in the masala for a further 5 mins. Cook for 2 more mins.

- Add some salt to taste & garam masala, to finish.

5. Tofu Tzatziki

Prep Time: 5 Mins, Total Time: 10 Mins, Serves: 4, Skill: Easy

Ingredients

- A pinch pepper
- Extra-firm tofu 250g (drained)
- A pinch salt
- Extra virgin olive oil 2 tbsp.
- Garlic cloves 2
- Chopped mint 1 tbsp.
- Juice from 1/2 a lemon
- Cucumber ½

Directions

- Blitz all the ingredients in the blender, except the cucumber, till smooth.
- Chop the cucumber in half & scratch the seeds out (the watery part) (the watery part)
- Grate the remainder of the cucumber & stir it to the mixture.
- Serve & enjoy.

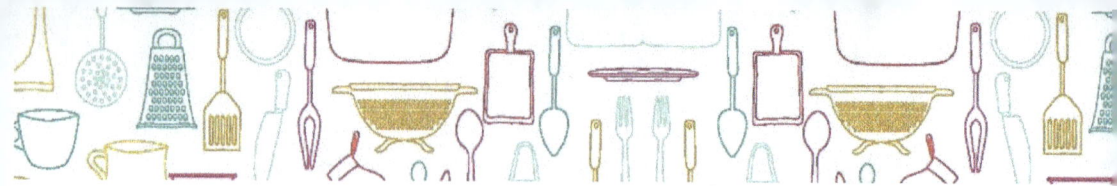

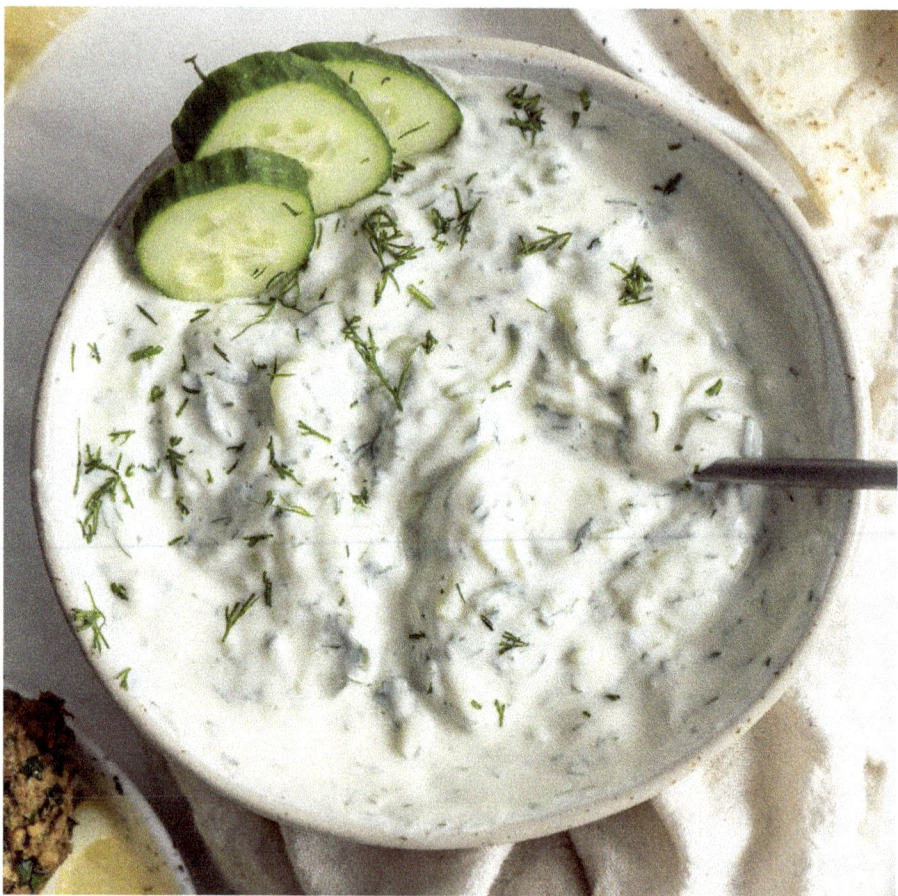

6. Cinnamon Almond Butter Shake

Prep Time: 1 Min, Total Time: 5 Mins, Serves: 4, Skill: Easy

Ingredients

- Collagen peptides 1 scoop

- Unsweetened nut milk 1 1/2 cups

- Almond butter 2 tbsp.

- Cinnamon ½ tsp

- Golden flax meal 2 tbsp.

- Liquid stevia 15 drops

- Ice cubes 6–8

- Almond extract 1/8 tsp

- Salt 1/8 tsp

Directions

- In your blender, add the ingredients and blend into the smoothie setting.

- Pour and enjoy in a glass.

7. Tropical Mango and Pineapple Smoothie

Prep Time: 5 Mins, Total Time: 5 Mins, Serves: 2, Skill: Easy

Ingredients

- Water or almond milk 200ml

- Mango 180g

- Ice cubes 6-8

- Pineapple 160g

- Frozen banana 1/2

Directions

- In your blender, add the ingredients and blend into the smoothie setting.

- Pour and enjoy in a glass

8. Low-Carb Blueberry Protein Power Smoothie

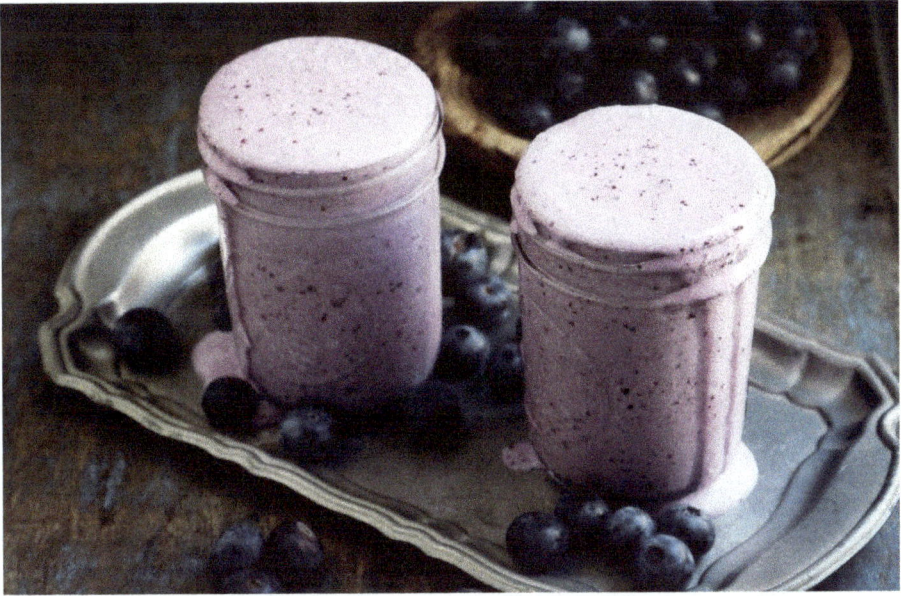

Prep Time: 2 Mins, Total Time: 5 Mins, Serves: 4, Skill: Easy

Ingredients

- Flaxseed meal **1 tbsp.**

- Fresh blueberries ¼ cup

- Simple syrup low carb, optional

- Unsweetened almond milk 8 oz.

- Vanilla whey protein 1 scoop

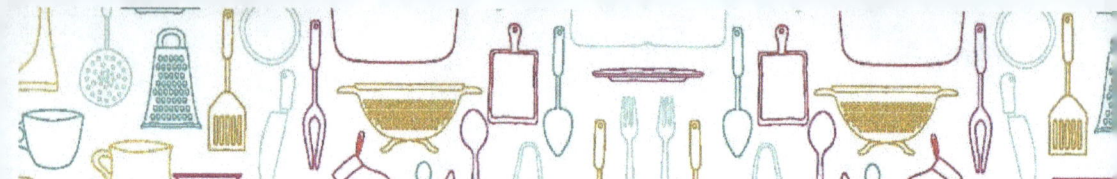

Directions

- Add all of the ingredients to the blender cup & use the smoothie option to blend.

- For a more filling meal, pour in a bowl or glass topped with more nuts, fruit, & granola.

9. Low-Carb 5 Minute Mocha Smoothie

Prep Time: 3 Mins, Total Time: 5 Mins, Serves: 4, Skill: Easy

Ingredients

- Coconut milk 1/2 cup

- Vanilla extract 1 teaspoon

- Unsweetened almond milk 1 1/2 cup

- Instant coffee 2 teaspoons

- Granulated erythritol/stevia blend 3 tablespoons

- Unsweetened cocoa powder 3 tablespoons

- Avocado 1 with pit removed cut in half

Directions

- Add all of the ingredients to the blender cup & use the smoothie option to blend.

- For a more filling meal, pour in a bowl or glass topped with more nuts, fruit, & granola.

10. Eggnog

Prep Time: 5 Mins, Total Time: 35 Mins, Serves: 4, Skill: Medium

Ingredients

- Seeds from vanilla pod 1

- Egg yolks 6

- Sweetened condensed milk 1 tin (397g)

- Spiced rum 150ml

- Heavy cream 1 tin (200g)

- 250ml milk

Directions

- Add to the blender jug all ingredients excluding rum

- Secure the lid & choose the PULSE feature to bring all the ingredients together.

- Choose SAUTE

- Upon completion of cooking, run the mixture through with a strainer to remove any lumps if necessary.

- Stir in some rum

- Both warm and chilled, serve

Chapter 5: Desserts

The dessert is the icing on the top of your mains and the Ninja is a must-try machine if you are a dessert lover. Below are some very scrumptious recipes for all sweet lovers. Give it a go and you will fall in love with the machine.

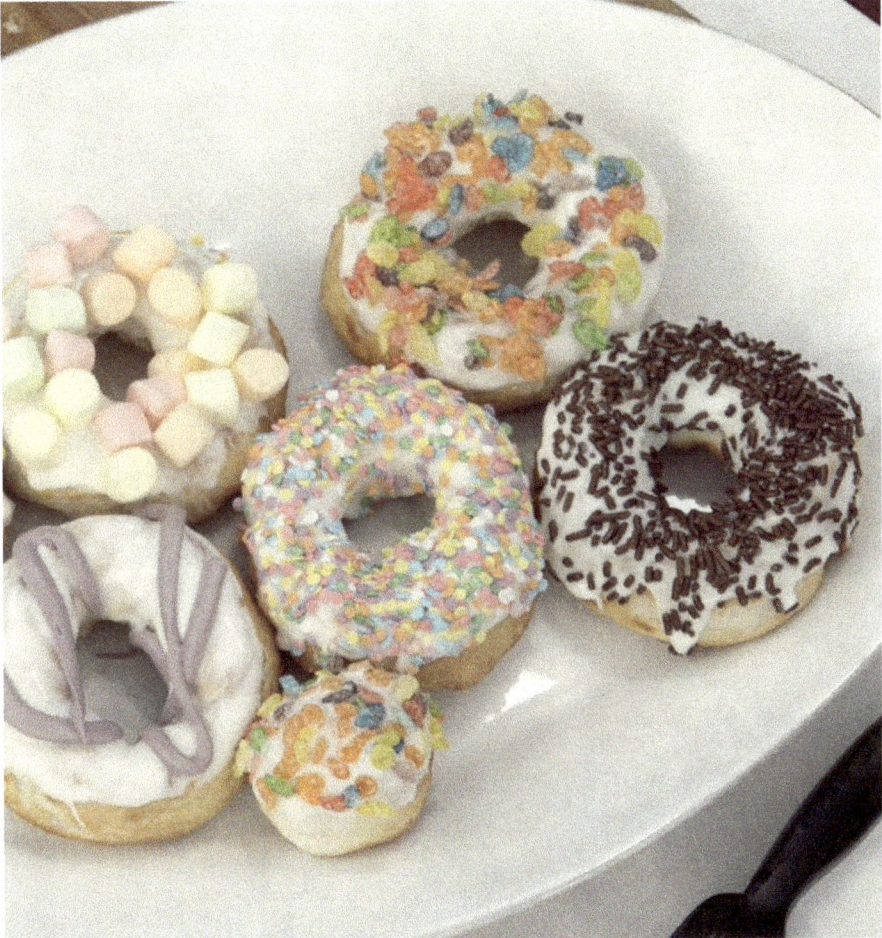

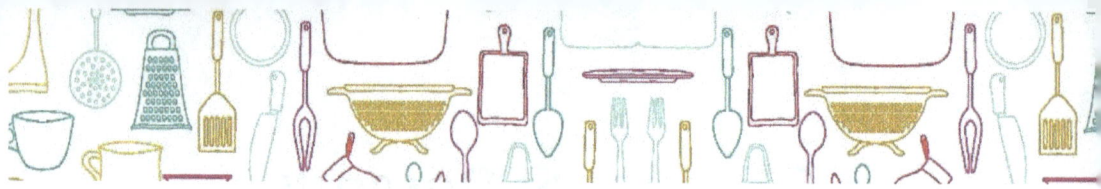

1. Raspberry and Chocolate Soup

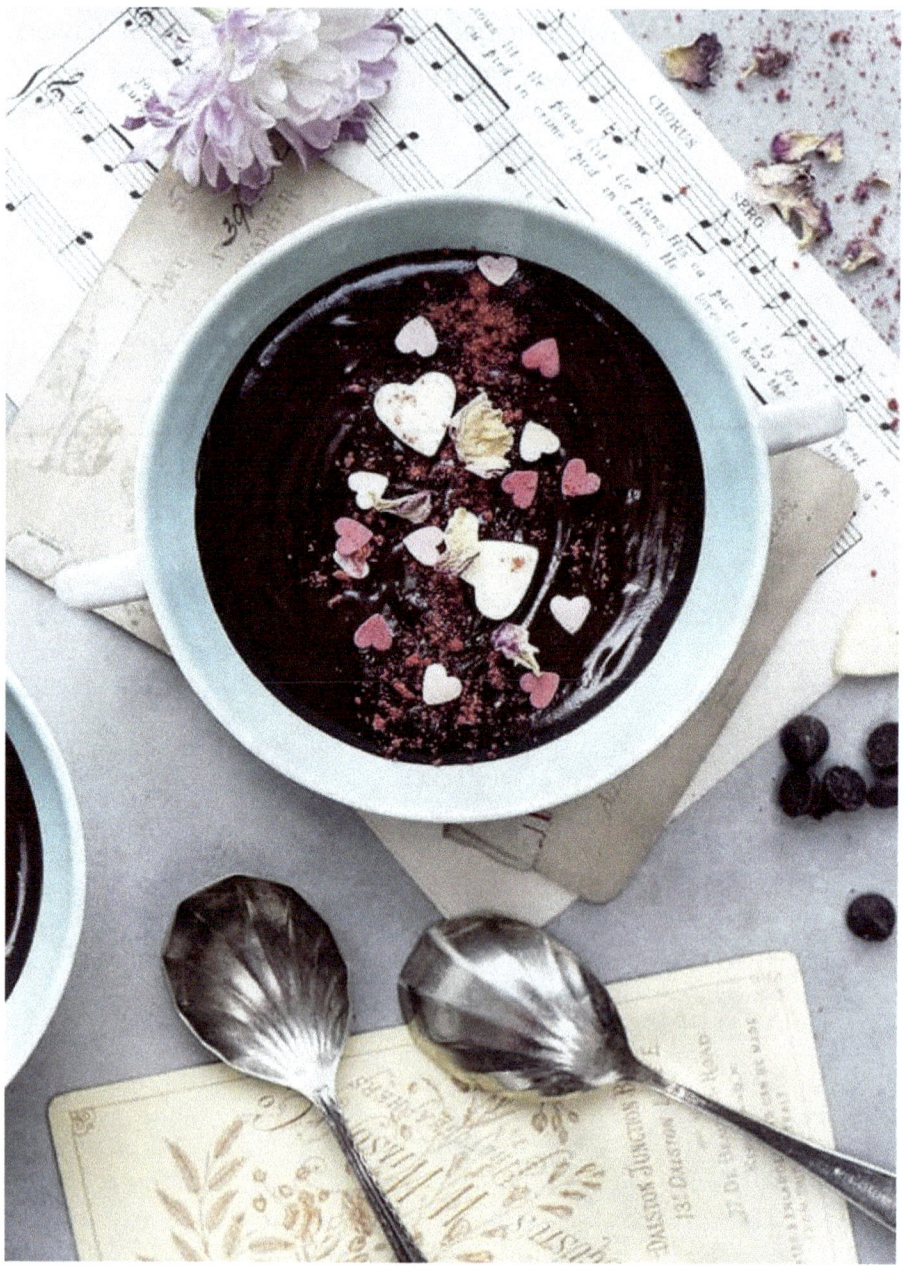

Prep Time: 2 Mins, Total Time: 35 Mins, Serves: 3, Skill: Medium

Ingredients

- Sea salt

- Full-fat coconut milk 1 can

- Vanilla extract 2 tsp

- Cold filtered water 250ml

- Frozen raspberries 200g

- Dark chocolate 50g

- Maple syrup 60ml

Directions

- To the pitcher of glass, insert all the ingredients. Close the lid & choose the configuration for the 'SMOOTH SOUP' & let the application run. Remove the lid cautiously after the application is finished and allow to cool for around 5 mins.

- In order to extract some raspberry seeds & serve instantly, push the soup via a coarse mesh sieve. Frozen raspberries, a spoonful of coconut yogurt, or chocolate curls are added to the top.

2. Peanut Butter Bombs

Prep Time: 10 Mins, Total Time: 40 Mins, Serves: 4, Skill: Medium

Ingredients

- A pinch of Salt

- Oats 150g

- Almond milk 4 tbsp.

- Peanut butter 3 tbsp.

- Melted coconut oil 1 tbsp.

- Maple syrup 3 tbsp.

For topping

- Chopped toasted peanuts 50g

- Dark chocolate 30g

Directions

- Insert the oats to the food processor & blend once flour develops.

- Add the rest of the ingredients (except the ingredients for topping) & blend again into a mixture that is sticky.

- Roll the combination into balls of similar size and position on a tray or plate.

- Melt the dark chocolate & drizzle over each ball at the top, a bit, finishing with a sprinkle of chopped nuts.

- Probably put 30 mins in the refrigerator to set

- Serve & enjoy. Make sure you carry it in an airtight jar & enjoy it for a week.

3. Sugar-Free Berry Sorbet

Prep Time: 5 Mins, Total Time: 65 Mins, Serves: 4, Skill: Medium

Ingredients

- A pinch of sea salt

- Frozen raspberries 350g

- Coconut water 215ml plus 2 tbsp.

- Frozen strawberries 150g

Directions

- In the Ninja Pitcher, put all the ingredients, lock the lid and choose 'ICE CREAM'. Run the application, scrub down the sides & repeat until completely combined & smooth, another 2 to 3 times.

- Shift to a container that is freezer-safe & airtight & freeze until firm for an hour. Serve with chocolate curls, fresh raspberries & desiccated coconut.

4. Banana Bread Granola

Prep Time: 5 Mins, Total Time: 25 Mins, Serves: 4, Skill: Easy

Ingredients

- Vanilla extract 1 tsp

- Jumbo oats 200g

- Cinnamon powder 1 tsp

- Bananas 2

- Coconut oil 1 tbsp.

- Chopped walnuts 60g

- Pinch of salt

- Maple syrup 3 tbsp.

Directions

- In a mixing bowl, mix the oats, cinnamon, walnuts, extract of vanilla, and a bit of salt.

- To the food processor, add the maple syrup, banana & coconut oil and process until smooth.

- Pour this mixture that is smooth with the dried ingredients into the bowl and blend properly.

- Line a tray for baking & spread the mixture of granola on it with baking paper. Assure it's very well packed, it will help make tasty crunchy granola clusters.

- Bake for about 20 minutes in the oven, or until golden. Enable it to cool entirely before removing it from the tray for baking.

5. Smooth Peanut and Almond Butter

Prep Time: 2 Mins, Total Time: 35 Mins, Serves: 10, Skill: Medium

Ingredients
- Mixed almonds & peanuts 525g

- Salt (optional)

Directions
- Insert the nuts & sprinkle with salt on a tray of baking.

- Bake for 10 mins at 160 degrees C /Gas Mark 3

- Enable to cool, then move to the food processor & process in quick bursts to ensure that you constantly scrape the sides off (It is best to process for around 15 mins & take short breaks in b/w).

- If required, taste & add salt.

- Store until ready to be used in the fridge.

6. Banana, Chia Seed & Peanut Butter Smoothie

Prep Time: 5 Mins, Total Time: 5 Mins, Serves: 4, Skill: Easy

INGREDIENTS

- Medium-sized ripe bananas 2

- Almond milk 750ml

- Linseeds 1 tbsp.

- Smooth peanut butter 2 tbsp.

- Chia seeds 2 tbsp.

Directions

- Put all the ingredients of the smoothie into the jug & blitz until smooth, utilizing the jug from the Ninja Kitchen System.

- Before serving, store in the refrigerator to cool

- Serve it cold & have fun.

7. Peanut Butter & Ingredient Banana Milkshake

Prep Time: 5 Mins, Total Time: 6 Mins, Serves: 2, Skill: Easy

Ingredients

- Almond milk 150ml

- Banana 1 (preferably frozen)

- Vanilla extract A dash (optional)

- Peanut butter 1 tbsp.

Directions

- Put all the ingredients of in the jug & blitz until smooth, using the Ninja Kitchen System.

- Before serving, store in the refrigerator to cool.

- Serve it cold & have fun.

8. Healthy Blueberry Slushies

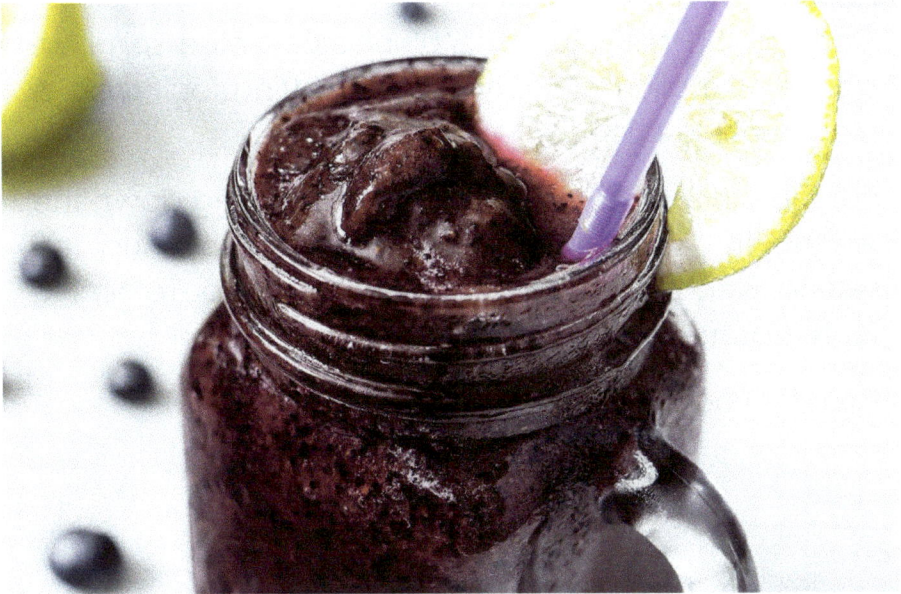

Prep Time: 1 Min, Total Time: 5 Mins, Serves: 4, Skill: Easy

Ingredients

- Ice 3 cups

- Frozen blueberries 2 cups

- Malic acid 1/2 tsp

- Light agave maple /nectar syrup 2-3 tbsp.

- Blue spirulina 2 tsp

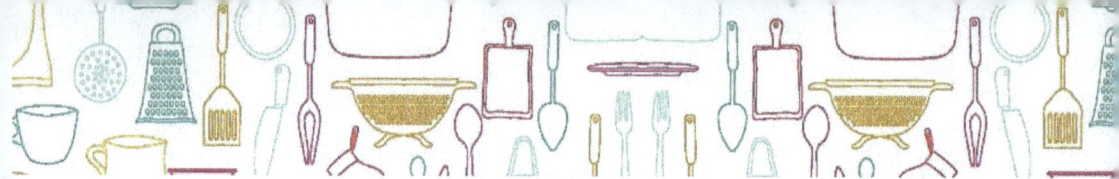

Directions

- Place in the Ninja jug; the blueberries, blue spirulina, agave, & malic acid. Choose the setting for 'Puree' & blend until smooth.

- Put the ice & choose 'Frozen drinks'. To bring down the ice on the sides, pause halfway and continue the setting. Blend repeatedly until the texture you're aiming for is reached.

- Pour for yourself into glasses & enjoy.

11. Kiwi and Lime Smoothie

Prep Time: 3 Mins, Total Time: 3 Mins, Serves: 1, Skill: Easy

Ingredients

- Protein powder 25g

- Coconut milk 200ml

- A handful of spinach

- Frozen banana 1

- Zest of lime 1

- Kiwi 1

Directions

- Add all of the ingredients to the blender cup & use the smoothie option to blend.

- For a more filling meal, pour in a bowl or glass topped with more nuts, fruit, & granola.

12. Homemade Panko Breadcrumbs

Prep Time: 5 Mins, Total Time: 20 Mins, Serves: 4, Skill: Easy

Ingredients

- White loaf small 1 (400g)

Directions

- Break off the bread crusts. Grate or put in a blender or food processor and pulse until chunky breadcrumbs are broken into

- Oven tray with parchment paper on the line. Arrange a single layer of breadcrumbs on parchment. ON Unit Transform. Choose BAKE, set a temperature of 140 °C, and set a time of 12 minutes. To commence preheating, click START / STOP

- Place the tray in the oven once the machine has pre-heated. Bake for 12 min, stirring once or twice with the breadcrumbs. Ensure that the breadcrumbs are crisp, or bake them for some minutes.

- It can be left to dry out in an open door oven.

- Store in an air-tight jar for up to 1 month until completely cooled.

13. Onion and Fig Jam

Prep Time: 5 Mins, Total Time: 45 Mins, Serves: 2, Skill: Medium

Ingredients

- Port wine 4 tbsp.

- Red onions 180g, cut into 4

- Pectin 30g

- Sugar 300g

- Butter 10g

- Cinnamon 1/2 tbsp.

- Cleaned figs 400g

- Ground ginger 1/2 tbsp.

Directions

- Switch on the heating blender, then pick SAUTE and COOK. Place the butter, sugar, 50g, and the onion in it. For 10 minutes, let the onions sauté, press the pulse key once, and then chop the others a little bit.

- Connect all other ingredients & use JAM to program your Blender.

- Pour the still-hot jam into two previously washed and sterilized jars after 30 minutes.

- As the jam cools down, close the jars & put them upright on their lids.

- When opened, keep a jam away from the hot weather or in the refrigerator.

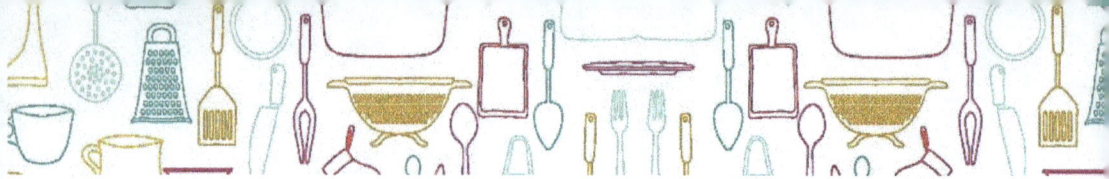

Serve with foie grass or game.

COOKING CONVERSION CHART

Measurement

CUP	ONCES	MILLILITERS	TABLESPOONS
8 cup	64 oz	1895 ml	128
6 cup	48 oz	1420 ml	96
5 cup	40 oz	1180 ml	80
4 cup	32 oz	960 ml	64
2 cup	16 oz	480 ml	32
1 cup	8 oz	240 ml	16
3/4 cup	6 oz	177 ml	12
2/3 cup	5 oz	158 ml	11
1/2 cup	4 oz	118 ml	8
3/8 cup	3 oz	90 ml	6
1/3 cup	2.5 oz	79 ml	5.5
1/4 cup	2 oz	59 ml	4
1/8 cup	1 oz	30 ml	3
1/16 cup	1/2 oz	15 ml	1

Temperature

FAHRENHEIT	CELSIUS
100 °F	37 °C
150 °F	65 °C
200 °F	93 °C
250 °F	121 °C
300 °F	150 °C
325 °F	160 °C
350 °F	180 °C
375 °F	190 °C
400 °F	200 °C
425 °F	220 °C
450 °F	230 °C
500 °F	260 °C
525 °F	274 °C
550 °F	288 °C

Weight

IMPERIAL	METRIC
1/2 oz	15 g
1 oz	29 g
2 oz	57 g
3 oz	85 g
4 oz	113 g
5 oz	141 g
6 oz	170 g
8 oz	227 g
10 oz	283 g
12 oz	340 g
13 oz	369 g
14 oz	397 g
15 oz	425 g
1 lb	453 g

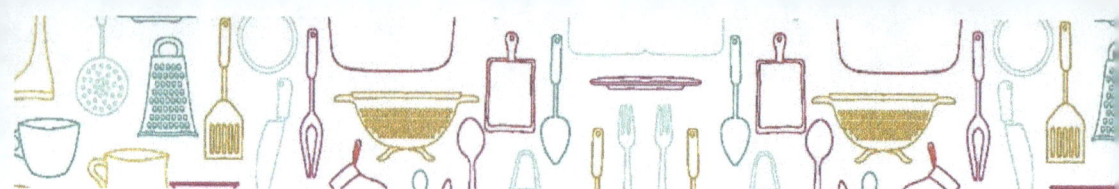

Conclusion

This was the marvelous world of cuisine with Ninja, which blends a pressure cooker's pace with an air fryer's quick-crisping operation. You can optimize your all-in-one system with this Complete Cookbook, by whipping uploads of quick, flavorful recipes.

This extensive cookbook provides everything one needs to start serving tasty, healthy recipes in minutes, from fish to Grill Baby Back Ribs. No matter what mood you are in, the Beginners Ninja Full Cookbook has what you want.

With the Cookbook for Beginners, bring mouth-watering meals to the table in no time. Not only you will learn a bundle of easy-to-cook recipes but you are also in for how to handle this astonishing state of the art device. It not only saves you time but also helps you in doing things in more perfect ways.

Soon you'll be the star in your family because of all these delicious, savory, and mouthwatering recipes. There is no need to waste your time grab your copies and start away and if you don't have the Foodi, then get it first.

CPSIA information can be obtained
at www.ICGtesting.com
Printed in the USA
BVHW091536180321
602886BV00003B/369

9 781802 230178